A Phenomenological Study of Depression in Iran

Moujan Mirdamadi

A Phenomenological Study of Depression in Iran

palgrave
macmillan

Moujan Mirdamadi
Prague, Czech Republic

ISBN 978-3-031-30406-4   ISBN 978-3-031-30407-1 (eBook)
https://doi.org/10.1007/978-3-031-30407-1

Cover illustration: © Alex Linch shutterstock.com

This Palgrave Macmillan imprint is published by the registered company Springer Nature Switzerland AG.
The registered company address is: Gewerbestrasse 11, 6330 Cham, Switzerland

Acknowledgements

I am grateful to many scholars, peers, and friends who have helped in the completion of this work. I thank my doctoral supervisors Rachel Cooper and Cain Todd, who guided me through this research. I am grateful for the constructive feedback from my colleagues at Lancaster University's Politics, Philosophy and Religion department, Hane Maung, Dan Degerman, Sam Fellows, and Brian Garvey, among others. I also thank Lancaster University's Faculty of Arts and Social Sciences for its financial support, which made this research possible.

The depth and breadth of this research was made possible through conversations I have been lucky to have with various scholars with varying expertise. I especially thank Joel Krueger, Matthew Ratcliffe, Benedict Smith, Orkideh Behrouzan, Mohsen Ashtiany, Houra Yavari, Jennifer Radden, and Jake Jackson for their constructive comments and suggestions at different stages of this research.

I would like to extend my gratitude to the staff at the Department of Psychiatry at University of Shiraz who helped in the acquisition of the empirical data presented in this work, in particular Dr Ebrahim Moghimi and Sepideh Ghorbani, who distributed the questionnaire among patients at Hafez University Clinic.

Lastly, I would like to thank Mehrdad Mirdamadi, for his unconditional support throughout this research. His emotional support and advice, especially with his knowledge of Iranian culture, has been invaluable and I greatly appreciate it.

Contents

List of Figures

1

Introduction

Depression, as one of the most common psychiatric disorders, has been subject to various studies and investigations. Different scholars have examined different aspects of depression—as a psychiatric classification, as lived illness experience, and as clusters of symptoms emphasised to different extents in different cultural contexts. The aim of the present work is to investigate the cultural shaping of depression and examine to what extent, if at all, experiences of depression as a psychiatric disorder can be traced to cultural scripts tied to specific sociocultural contexts. I offer a phenomenological analysis of depression, with first-person reports of experiences of depression as the starting point. Similar studies of mental disorders, concerned with the nature of individual experiences, have proved fruitful and informative and indeed form the background to the present investigation. Yet I hope to offer a novel approach in the phenomenological analysis by situating individual reports within a cultural context through which the meaning and significance of the self-reports can be discerned. In this sense, the links between cultural modes of understanding and interpretation, reflected in personal reports and narratives of depression, and the way depression is experienced and made sense of, can be brought to light. Such an account of depression has a considerable potential to go beyond the well-documented cross-cultural

M. Mirdamadi, *A Phenomenological Study of Depression in Iran*,
https://doi.org/10.1007/978-3-031-30407-1_1

variations in manifestation of mental disorders, instead offering insight into how the link between culture and illness experience and expression ought to be understood.

The investigation adopts a comparative approach by taking first-person accounts of depression previously gathered in the UK, alongside those collected in Iran in the course of this research. The considerable differences in the cultural norms, beliefs, and values of the two countries, presents a case where similarities in reports of experiences of depression can attest to the universality of symptoms and nature of experiences. On the other hand, for the same reason, variations in experiences of depression could be plausibly traced and accounted for within the specific cultural context. As I will show, levels of religiosity, the place of individuality in the culture, as well as historical experiences and changes are among factors that can reasonably be linked with current conceptualisations and experiences of depression. By viewing the individual as an agent situated within a particular sociocultural context, a dynamic relation is established whereby the dominant frameworks for understanding and interpretation influence an individual's perception and experiences of the illness, while the depressed individual navigates the cultural landscapes by creating her own narratives and interpretations of her experience.

Various studies have established the fact of the presence of variations in manifestations of depression across cultures. Some of the earlier research can be understood as making broad comparisons between western and eastern experiences and manifestations of depression (e.g. Kleinman 1982, 1986), while some of the later ones have focused on specific symptoms which present differently in different cultures (Haroz et al. 2016) resulting in different help-seeking behaviours (e.g. Naeem et al. 2012; Ying 1990; Ying et al. 2000). The significance of these investigations and findings, predominantly in the fields of medical anthropology and cross-cultural psychiatry, is made clear against the background of the mostly universalist and western-centric approach to psychiatric classifications. These approaches, best exemplified by the *Diagnostic and Statistical Manual of Mental Disorders* (DSM), view disorders and their symptoms as largely universal and shaped independently of culture. This universalist approach has had a considerable role in making psychiatric classifications and diagnostic criteria accessible in different cultures and settings. Yet it tends to assign to culture only a marginal influence on manifestation and expression of disorders. This tendency remains largely intact despite some changes brought about as a result of scholarly work highlighting the important role of culture in shaping some disorders such as depression.

Importantly, although within the body of scholarly work on the topic the importance of culture in shaping manifestations and articulations of depression is highlighted, there remains a lack of in-depth investigations into the different ways in which culture can be shown to shape experiences of depression. In particular, the dynamics by which the cultural modes of thought and interpretation influence the individual experiences of depression, as situated within a given sociocultural context, remain largely overlooked. This gap is the motivation for the present phenomenological analysis, which not only focuses on depression as it is conceptualised and experienced by those suffering from the disorder, but also views the individual as an agent situated within a particular sociocultural context. Such an investigation, therefore, attempts to go beyond the individual experiences by identifying different ways in which, culture as a system of interpretation and meaning making, shapes and moulds experiences and understandings of depression. It is not just the *fact* of variation in manifestation of symptoms across cultures that is of interest, but rather the question of *how* these variations are rooted in cultural contexts, and *how* they ought to be made sense of against a sociocultural background within which experiences and narratives are situated.

The particular focus and interest of the present study means it diverges from the recent phenomenological interest in mental disorders, while being firmly rooted in them. Phenomenologists are largely concerned with universal structures of our consciousness, which is assumed to be common to all individuals, regardless of their cultural and social backgrounds. There has therefore been little room for phenomenological investigations in light of culture and cultural variation. Thus, a key point I aim to demonstrate in this work is that phenomenology can, and ought to view individual conscious experiences as situated within a sociocultural context that gives these experiences their significance and meaning.

Despite this divergence, the present study has been made possible by other phenomenological investigations of depression, most notably, Matthew Ratcliffe's *Experiences of Depression: A study in phenomenology* (2015). Ratcliffe offers a systematic phenomenological account of depression based upon first-person accounts from a qualitative questionnaire, works of literature and memoirs. This analysis of the existential changes involved in the experiences of depression and the various aspects of individual understanding of the world and things within it offer invaluable insight into the world of depression. By viewing the qualitative data in Ratcliffe's investigation alongside those collected in Iran, a new layer of analysis emerges: one that gives centre-stage to sociocultural norms, customs and conceptions shaping individual experiences and understandings of depression. This new depth of analysis enables a cross-cultural account of variations in experiences of depression through an exposition of the cultural context and background, which give meaning and significance to the experiences, as the subject of the phenomenological enquiry. What emerges is a sketch of the different ways in which culture can be shown to underlie the variations in experiences and understandings of depression, thus giving a broader, more accurate understanding of depression as an illness category.

Methodology

The present work is informed by first-person accounts of depression, tokens of which are presented throughout the analysis as numbered quotes. These were collected in two parts: firstly, through collection of public posts on Facebook; and secondly through an open-ended questionnaire. These personal accounts and narratives of depression offer an insight into common themes of experiences and complaints among Iranian depressed patients which can be traced and accounted for through appeal to longstanding cultural concepts and frameworks.

Personal accounts posted on Facebook followed an open invitation during the mental health awareness week in April 2015, encouraging open conversation about depression to combat misconceptions and stigma around the disorder in Iranian society. The result was first, a considerable number of individuals taking to Facebook to express and talk about what they understood to be the most important elements of their experience of depression, and later on the creation of a Facebook support group for Iranians suffering from depression. Around 20 of these accounts were posted publicly, and shared widely for public reading. These are included in the analysis and marked with 'FB' in text.

Themes identified in the Facebook accounts were used to inform the questionnaire which aimed to acquire more targeted personal accounts of depression. Following the format of the questionnaire conducted by Ratcliffe and colleagues at Durham University (Ratcliffe 2015), the depression questionnaire comprised of open-ended questions with no limits on the length of responses, and thus prompted respondents to give detailed accounts of different aspects of their experiences of depression (see appendix). Despite attempts at conducting the questionnaire solely online, by posting it on different forums and support groups focused on depression, no more than 10 participants took part online.[1] Through collaboration with practitioners and psychiatrists in the country, the questionnaire was also distributed in an out-patient psychiatric clinic in Shiraz,[2] yielding an additional 33 responses. The 43 total responses are the main source of data for the present analysis and the numbered quotes in the text are taken from this pool of questionnaire responses; both online and from the clinic. As will be seen in the following chapters, these are analysed and made sense of alongside the Facebook posts, and situated within a range of cultural resources to facilitate a more comprehensive analysis.

The questionnaire conducted in Iran has three additional questions compared to the one conducted in the UK. These were added following

[1] Reasons for this could include a lack of trust among individuals for sharing their experiences with a stranger (arguably heightened by the lack of independent institutions and free research in the country); lack of access to the internet and widespread censorship of online spaces, among others. Such background elements should nonetheless be borne in mind as limitations faced by such research in a country with different norms and conditions concerning qualitative research, especially in the absence of researcher.

[2] I would like to thank Dr Ebrahim Moghimi and Ms Sepideh Ghorbani for their help facilitating this part of the research.

the preliminary analysis of Facebook accounts, and aimed to explore in more depth particular elements talked about by Iranians. Two of these reflect the heavy emphasis placed on interpersonal relations as shaping experiences of depression among Iranians. The third reflects previous research that identifies sadness and dysphoria as central characteristics of depression in Iran.

- How would you describe your relationships with others when you are depressed?
- Has the reaction of others influenced your experience of depression? If so, how?
- What distinguishes what you're feeling as depression, from other, more general forms of sadness?[3]

The questionnaire responses were used to identify common themes in experiences of depression in Iran that were indicative of variation when compared against the UK sample, either in type, manifestation, or degree of emphasis.[4] These themes (Fig. 1.1) have been analysed and accounted for through various theories within the phenomenological literature, as well as works in anthropology, sociology, and psychology, where these provide a framework for discerning the phenomenological and cultural significance of the variations. In all instances, in order to situate the experiences and complaints in a culturally significant context, I outline the relevant sociocultural and historical elements unique to the Iranian ethos, which can be shown to have phenomenological significance, through their influence in shaping the experiences of depression as expressed in the responses. Each of these themes of variation, are the subject of different chapters in the work, together with the corresponding phenomenological analyses of their significance against a particular sociocultural element.

---

[3] I thank Dr Benedict Smith for his suggestion of the question clarifying the distinction between depression and other forms of sadness in Iran.

[4] It should be noted that in conducting the comparative element with the UK sample, I refer only to the published material from the Durham study and not to any part of the raw data associated with it.

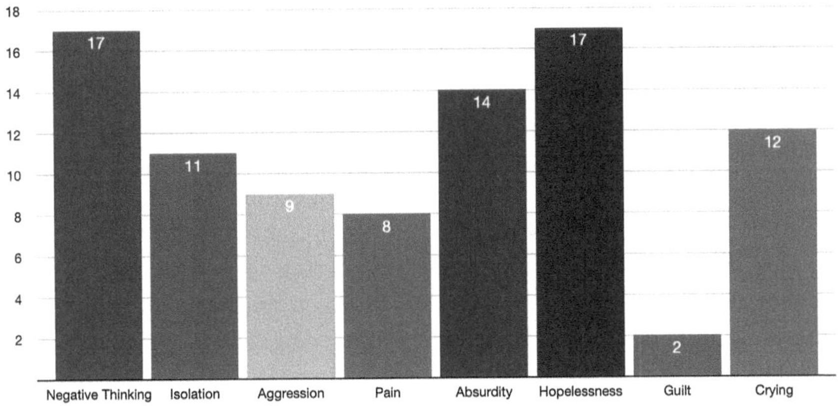

Fig. 1.1 Common symptom reports among Iranian patients

As I note in the following chapters, Iranian population is made up of various ethnic, religious and linguistic groups which attest to the heterogeneity of experiences of depression. Results of this study, therefore, given the sample size but also its mode of conduct—presented only in the official language Farsi and reliant on access to the internet or a psychiatric clinic—are not to be taken as representative of all experiences of depression in the country. Instead, the aim of the present investigation has been to identify common themes in experiences of depression which can be made sense of, through examination of cultural elements shared among the majority of this heterogenous population. In other words, the personal accounts are used alongside cultural conceptions to offer a plausible account of the ways in which culture can shape experiences of depression by constructing a meaning-making context for experiences. It should also be noted that differences in norms and concerns in research in Iran, together with broad restrictions that often hinder independent academic investigations, mean reproducing research methods in Iran is often unlikely. For instance, the lack of popular free access to online content in the country clearly limits any method reliant on online platforms. For these reasons, it is important to make explicit what is implied throughout this work—namely, that I do not claim to present here a generalised image of how depression is felt and experienced in Iran, but rather, to offer a way in which culture can be shown to underly certain experiences and manifestations of depression that are varied in different sociocultural contexts.

Lastly, a worry should also be noted here regarding the epistemic reliability of the responses to the questionnaire. It is conceivable that the profound existential change involved in depression would be reflected in self-reports of experiences, bringing to question the accuracy and reliability of the report. Whilst I acknowledge this possibility, I do not view it as a problem for the purposes of this study. For part of the investigation here is precisely the ways in which one's understanding and interpretation of one's daily experiences (e.g. relations with, and perceptions of others) are changed in the course of depression, and how these changes are articulated by individuals in depression. As such, responses to the questionnaire are informative of experiences and individuals' understandings of them, regardless of how accurately and reliably they represent the individual's experiences.

Chapter Outline and Summary of Argument

As noted earlier, the analysis presented in the book is divided based on the identified themes, where each chapter looks at a different cluster of symptoms that can be analysed together. Chapter 2 precedes the main analysis by providing the broad context and background against which the analysis is carried out. The elements discussed in this chapter form the foundation of the later discussions, in giving accounts of the role culture plays in shaping experiences of depression. In addition to giving a broad sketch of the sociocultural make-up of Iran, an overview of historical events which have significantly influenced the dominant discourse and culture of Iran today is given. I will also give a brief exposition of the history of psychiatry in Iran, showing how the trajectory of pedagogical and practical psychiatry has progressed in light of historical and cultural changes in the country. This history is important in understanding conceptions of psychiatry among the public, and the expectations that result from such conceptions. This exposition is followed by a sketch of the various cultural elements that shape the Iranian conception of depression in particular. I argue that the dominant understanding of depression among Iranians is heavily influenced by (a) traditional Iranian and Islamic medicine, which have shaped folk beliefs around health, illness and medicine, (b) character types that Iranians aspire to, how individuals view themselves and others in light of these ideals, and (c) the cultural modes of causal attributions. Using examples from responses to the questionnaire, I show how these elements all play a role in the dominant ways of conceptualising depression. In the last section, drawing on previous research on Iran, I offer a way of understanding the place of sadness and dysphoria in Iranian culture. Crucially, I argue, contrary to previous studies, that such emotions rather than being valued and emphasised in their own right, draw their place in the culture following the long-standing cultural conceptions of life, as a fight between forces of Good and Evil. As I will show in later chapters, this way of viewing life has important consequences for the understanding and interpretation of experiences of depression in Iran.

In Chap. 3 I will look at metaphors used in descriptions of depression experiences, as a form of narrative that can offer important insights into the way depression is conceptualised, experienced and articulated. Using the cognitive-linguistic theory of metaphors, I examine the implications of the variation in the use of metaphors in different cultures for understanding experiences themselves. In particular, I will look at two sets of metaphors used by Iranians in describing their experiences, showing that while some might be reducible to universal metaphors used in other cultures, others arise from culturally specific conceptions and experiences. By tracing the use and significance of such metaphors to important literary works and cultural conceptions, I argue that metaphors carry within them important insights into cultural ways of understanding and encountering depression. In the case of Iran, such metaphors express the dominant ways of viewing the world in depression, as well as the cultural conceptions of depression itself.

In Chap. 4, I give an explanation for the presence of a sense of absurdity among Iranian depressed patients, as well as for the variation in the emphasis placed on the feeling of hopelessness, and attitudes towards suicide. I argue that what links these variations together is the presence of a culture of death-consciousness in Iran, reflected in religious texts and works of literature, and amplified following the Iran-Iraq war and the dominant discourse around it. After giving an argument for the presence of this culture in Iran, manifested through these elements, and drawing on points noted in Chap. 2, I argue that the presence of absurdity and the stronger emphasis on hopelessness can be explained through cultural frameworks for thought and understanding found in Iran today.

Chapters 5 and 6 are concerned with the alterations in one's way of being with others in depression, and the variations in this domain between Iran and the UK. The discussion is divided into social relationships, particularly those between an individual and the society (Chap. 5), and interpersonal relationships between individuals (Chap. 6). Here, variations in emotional experiences in depression, arising from misunderstandings of depression prevalent in Iranian society, are accounted for through phenomenological and cultural considerations. I particularly look at issues of social stigmatisation of depression, empathy, absence of guilt and presence of aggression among Iranian patients, and the tendency towards isolation. Drawing on phenomenological literature, particularly those of Sartre and Heidegger, I highlight the interpersonal conflict central to two phenomenologists' accounts of relationships with others, to argue that in depression this conflict comes to the foreground of consciousness and determines one's experiences in these domains. The heightened perception of the conflict between one and others, together with the unique sociocultural context, can be shown to account for the variations in interpersonal experiences in depression.

Chapter 7 deals with the issue of somatisation in depression and aims to give an account of the significance of somatic symptoms and their variation cross-culturally. I draw on phenomenological literature on embodiment to argue that somatic symptoms ought to be understood as a constitutive part of the overall experience of depression universally, rather than a culturally specific element of experiences, as is often portrayed in the cross-cultural literature. Despite this universality, I argue that the manifestation and emphasis placed on different somatic symptoms varies across cultures. Taking the case of pain as one of the most complained about physical symptom among Iranian patients, and noting the cultural significance of pain, I offer an account for understanding the special emphasis placed on this symptom among Iranian patients.

In Chap. 8 I offer a theoretical framework for understanding the relationship between culture, experiences, and narratives of depression. Building on the arguments from the previous sections and drawing on literature in philosophy and anthropology, I argue for an understanding of experiences as inherently cultural, inseparable from the context in which they are had, and the narratives expressing and describing them. Through this theoretical understanding I build an argument against the notion of 'idioms of distress', widely used in cross-cultural studies of disorders. I argue that the notion lacks explanatory power and as such cannot be used to account for variations, for although it signals the fact of the presence of differences arising from cultural concepts, it does little by way of explaining why and how these differences come about.

In Chap. 9, I discuss the implications of the study for the science and practice of psychiatry, and for phenomenology as a discipline and method. As I claim, the arguments of the work have consequences for our understanding of pathological symptoms as well as disorders more broadly. Similarly, the need for sensitivity to culture as the background of all our conscious experiences and understanding of the world has implications for phenomenology as the study of structures of our human consciousness.

2

The Iranian Context

Iran is located on a 1.5 thousand square kilometre plateau, reaching in the North to the Caspian Sea, and in the South to the Persian Gulf and the Gulf of Oman, bordering Afghanistan and Pakistan in the East, and Iraq and Turkey in the West. According to the latest census conducted in 2015 the country had a population of just under 80 million; 59.1 million living in urban areas, compared to only 20.3 million living in villages and small towns. The urban population of Iran has been continuously growing in recent years, whilst smaller villages and towns have seen a reduction in population. The province of Fars, located in the south of the country, where the present study was conducted, is largely rural and has the highest share of nomadic population (*ashāyer*) in the country, including big nomadic communities and various nomadic clans. Despite being almost 10 times the land size of Tehran (population 13.3 million), Fars has a population of just under 5 million (Statistical Center of Iran 2015). The psychiatric clinic where outpatients were recruited for the questionnaire is located in the capital and largest city in the province, Shiraz, where patients from different parts of the province receive care.

M. Mirdamadi, *A Phenomenological Study of Depression in Iran*,
https://doi.org/10.1007/978-3-031-30407-1_2

Iran has a young population, with over 75% being aged forty or under, and over 21% aged between 25 and 34. Over half of the adult population have a high school diploma and/or have a higher education certificate. These statistics vary in different parts of Iran, due to the centralisation of wealth, jobs and education opportunities in larger cities especially Tehran. Yet the general picture of demographics and education levels highlights the changing nature of attitudes and beliefs in the culture to be covered in the later chapters.

According to the official statistics, 99.6% of Iranians identify as Muslims, with Christianity, Zoroastrianism, Judaism, and other 'undeclared' religions respectively forming the biggest religious minorities in the country. It is worth noting that the official statistics do not take into account different belief systems within a religion. Thus, although there is a Sunni minority in Iran, no official statistics exist on the proportions of Sunni and Shi'ite belief systems. Shi'ism is the official religion of the country and the state, and as the most widely held faith in the country, has had a large influence in the present sociocultural make-up of the country. It should be noted that Shi'ism as practiced in Iran differs in notable ways from other countries and cultures that practice this branch of Islam, such as Iraq and Syria. This difference is in part due to the official status of Shi'ism and its association with the ruling regime, which highlights and encourages certain teachings and customs of the belief system, and in part due to the influence of pre-Islamic culture of Iran (Persia), which has shaped the practice in the country to have its unique Iranian form.

Similarly, no official data is collected on ethnic and language minorities in the country. Although Persian ethnicity and language form the majority of the country (over 60%), there are various other languages and ethnic backgrounds which have had a considerable influence on the culture. The largest minority groups, both ethnic and linguistic, include Azeri (16%), Kurd (10%), Lur (6%), Baluch (2%) and Arab (2%) (Minority Rights Group International 2017).

Despite the large cultural diversity and heterogeneity of the country as demonstrated by the demographic data, the official status of Persian language and Shi'ite belief system give them an unparalleled influence in shaping cultural scripts and narratives. They therefore ought to be viewed as significant pillars of the culture throughout the analysis. Persian literature, in particular, has been a mirror of the Iranian culture and concerns of the society throughout history. One reason for this continued influence is the fact that the Persian language, as primarily a spoken language, flourished in the form of poetry, different instances of which continue to be used as everyday expressions. "For Iranians, poetry precedes literacy; it is carried 'in the chest', an expression indicating that Iranians' poetic heritage lives on from one generation to the next, in hearts and in memory, shaping part of the cultural aesthetics of the literate and illiterate alike" (Behrouzan 2016, p. 13). Despite the changes to the language itself over the years, pieces from literary works, and especially poetry remain a strong medium through which Iranians express their emotions and everyday concerns and preoccupations.

Furthermore, as the most dominant form of art in Iranian culture, Persian poetry and literature offer an insight into the social and political changes in Iranian society, especially in the modern era. In the absence of sustained scholarly research and institutions and given the history of expressiveness and influential power of poetry, this medium became, and remains, the one reflecting the goings on at the heart of the culture and society. Given this sustained influence, in addition to reflecting the dominant culture, Persian poetry and literature also offer an insight into how the thoughts and concerns of the Iranian people have changed and evolved throughout the years. The creation and popularity of different works of literature during political upheavals, and the censorship of different works under different ideological governments throughout history, show the historically important role of literature in reflecting the sociocultural changes of Iran.

The influential power of Shi'ism is especially seen through the discourse that has dominated Iran following the Islamic revolution of 1979, as it marks an enormous shift in value system and modes of conduct that have been enforced ever since. The new regime, in an attempt to distance itself from the monarchical Pahlavi dynasty that it had overthrown, reversed many of their policies and approaches to governance. The most important of these reversals that has changed the face of Iran ever since, was the enforcement of Islamic law in all domains of life. This 'Islamisation' of governance and public life in Iran has defined a powerful public discourse, which after almost 40 years, has had an undeniable influence on cultural modes of thought and understanding.

Another historical event that plays an important role in talking about Iranian culture as seen today is the Iran-Iraq war in the 1980s. The eight-year war had devastating effects in the country, which remain visible today, 30 years after the events. These effects include large areas close to the border which have never recovered from war, minefields that continue to take lives, as well as the continuing sense of loss for those who never found out the fate of their loved ones. During the war, Iran saw a population boom as well, following policy changes after the revolution. In a reversal of the previous regime's policy, the newly established government started promoting larger family sizes. With the start of the war, these promotions carried stronger emphasis, since a larger population was seen as an advantage in the war (Karamouzian et al. 2014, p. 231). The population boom resulting from such policies was such that a large part of the present population of Iran was either born, or had a large portion of their childhood spent during the war. The war also worked to cement the new Islamic and ideological discourse that continues to shape a large part of the Iranian psyche. These continuing effects of war and the shared generational memories of the events have a considerable impact on the way depression is conceptualised and experienced in Iran (see Behrouzan 2016).

History of Psychiatry in Iran

A brief history of psychiatric teachings in Iran will help a better understanding of the care for and conceptualisations of mental disorders in the country. As early as the nineteenth century AD, well-known names in Iranian and Islamic medicine, such as Avicenna (Ibn-Sina) and Rhazes (al-Razi), wrote about illnesses of the soul, such as melancholia, and how they can be remedied (Dols 1992). Although these discussions of mental illness have had their place in Iranian medical traditions, modern psychiatry in Iran began with the founding of University of Tehran in 1934, where the department of psychiatry began the formal education of students in the field a few years later.

Before the formalisation of psychiatric care, various asylums for the mentally ill could be found in Tehran and elsewhere around the country, known as *dārolmajānin*, or madhouses. These asylums, often managed by local authorities, and funded by charity endowments, often suffered from poor conditions (Javanbakht and Sanati 2006), and accommodated a range of criminal, poor, mentally impaired, and handicapped individuals (Behrouzan 2016). The asylums became the subject of various socially critical books and novels, that aimed to tell the stories of individuals in the asylums as well as the conditions under which they were kept and cared for (e.g. Ali Akbar Jamalzadeh's *Darolmajanin*, 1942).

Such asylums were repurposed into psychiatric wards and clinics when modern psychiatry came to Iran in the 1930s and 1940s. This arrival was due to waves of students who were sent abroad for education and training beginning from the 1930s. The first group of students who would later lay the foundations of psychiatric pedagogy in Iran (such as Ebrāhim Chehrāzi, Abdolhossein Mirsepāssi, and Hossein Rezaei), were trained in France. These French-educated founders were trained in neurology and neuropsychiatry and therefore had a largely biological orientation (Behrouzan 2016, p. 42). As Behrouzan notes, the distinction between *mental* and *nervous* diseases, which followed psychological and/or psychoanalytic traditions, and neurological sciences respectively, characterised the psychiatric education in Iran. This distinction was evidenced by the first teaching curricula, built by "a generation of scientific, Francophile, can-do modernizers" (Ibid., p. 49). It was during this time, in 1946, that Ruzbeh hospital, the first modern psychiatric teaching hospital, was built in Tehran, and it continues to be at the forefront of psychiatric care and education in the country.

The influence of psychoanalysis on psychiatric education and practice, was not seen in Iran until the 1970s. The Iranian public were introduced to some psychoanalytical concepts, through radio programmes (Behrouzan 2016, p. 50), and a few translations by non-specialists of some of Freud's works, in the 1950s (Barzin 2010). Despite this familiarity, the influence of Freud and his works remained largely outside the medical domain. This changed when another generation of foreign-educated students returned from the US, bringing with them a legacy of psychoanalysis, as a dominant force in American psychiatry at the time.

Psychoanalytic traditions had an influence both on the education of psychiatry, for instance at Ruzbeh, as well as in practice, with many of those oriented towards psychoanalytic traditions setting up private practices in Tehran and other larger cities such as Isfahan and Shiraz. Various research programmes in psychoanalytic research and training were formed, and along with biomedically focused programmes, they offered a mixed pedagogy of psychiatry at universities and hospitals.

The marriage of the two traditions ended with the Islamic revolution of 1979, when the ideological forces, and the public opinion which equated psychoanalysis "with unconsciousness, repression, resistance, libido and the irrational sexualization of everything" (Shoja Shafti 2005, p. 388), created unsavoury circumstances for practitioners and experts in psychoanalysis, causing many of the leading members to leave Iran or limit their influence to private practices. At this time, psychoanalytic teachings were abandoned and the focus was again shifted to biomedical orientations. Furthermore, during the Cultural Revolution of 1980–1983, which aimed at the 'cleansing' of academia, the focus of psychiatric practice, education, and discourse, shifted further to accommodate for the newly formed value system. Although there would be a renewed interest in psychoanalytic traditions in the late 1980s and 1990s, this was heavily influenced, and determined by a newly defined value system that education and practice would have to adhere to.

During the cultural revolution universities were closed for three years, during which time a large number of faculty staff, including some of those psychiatrists who pioneered psychoanalysis, either left or were dismissed (Behrouzan 2016, p. 52). Following the Cultural Revolution, although the broader medical curriculum remained largely unchanged, psychiatry "was implicitly neglected early on, if not disdained, as either a bourgeois discipline or as inconsequential compared to other medical specialities" (Ibid., p. 53). Eventually, however, with the war ending in the late 1980s and especially with the return of war veterans in need of psychiatric help, the importance of, and need for psychiatric care was recognised. This recognition resulted in a sense of pragmatism with respect to psychiatry, which allowed it to be practiced more or less freely, while psychiatric pedagogy became increasingly biomedical and psychopharmacologically oriented.

Given the large influence of the Revolution and the Iran-Iraq war, the psychiatric attitude that emerged in public discourse in the 1990s differed considerably from that of the late 1970s. This attitude was influenced by two elements. First was the concern with the implementation of religious codes of conduct and Shi'ite moral order in the society, as the new dominant moral and value system. Second was the concern with the wellbeing and care of those influenced by war, including veterans and prisoners of war, and their families, as well as the families of martyrs. It was within this context, and against the backdrop of increasingly biomedical psychiatric pedagogy, that the new emphasis on psychoanalytic traditions was formulated.

The new attention to psychoanalysis in Iran was largely pressed for by Mohammad San'ati, who was trained in the UK and returned to Iran in 1985. As one of the first psychiatrists to appear on radio and TV shows, San'ati advocated for attention to psychoanalysis not as an alternative to the biomedical traditions now firmly in place and widely supported, but as complementary to these traditions. Whilst navigating the public discourse with emphasis on clinical and medical models of psychiatry, San'ati brought psychoanalytic traditions into the public domain through his analyses of well-known Iranian literary works, while at the same time training students in psychoanalysis at his home (Behrouzan 2016, p. 57). Through his efforts, in 1996 a new curriculum was designed for teaching dynamic therapies to psychiatry residents, which led to the 2008 implementation of a residency curriculum that included 9-month training in dynamic psychotherapies. In 2014, a fellowship in analytical psychotherapy was launched at the Dynamic Psychotherapy and Human Studies Unit (itself established in 2006) at the University of Tehran.

Today, psychiatric education is more or less uniform across universities in Iran, due to the national standardisation of curricula. The curriculum in use currently is firmly situated within the biomedical tradition for understanding and treating mental disorders. Some of the broader topics in the curricula include: neuroscience and neurology, basics of human psychology, psychiatric classifications (ICD and DSM), clinical psychiatric assessments, and biomedical and pharmacological treatment options for psychiatric illnesses (Secretariat of Council for Medical and Specialised Education – Ministry of Health and Medical Education 2007). Training in psychotherapy is not a central element within this curriculum and any larger emphases on psychotherapy is dependent on the individual institutions; for instance at Ruzbeh hospital, the opportunity to study such topics in more detail is greater, as compared to other programmes in other parts of the country.

Currently, psychiatric diagnoses in Iran are based on the DSM-IV-TR[1] and the vast majority of treatment methods around the country are biomedical ones. Although centres for counselling can be found in different parts of Iran, psychotherapy and psychoanalysis remain scarce and mainly exclusive to Tehran. Due to the time-consuming nature of such treatments and their high cost compared to other treatment methods, the demand for these is limited to the more well-off parts of the population, which remain largely concentrated in Tehran. As Behrouzan notes, even for those clinicians and students who are interested, training in psychotherapy and psychodynamic traditions is often sacrificed for the financial security offered by biomedical and pharmacological practices, due to their high demand among the larger public. At the Hafez University Hospital in Shiraz, where the empirical part of the present research was conducted, the following services are offered for psychiatric patients: “medical therapy, shock therapy, occupational therapy, psychological counselling for individuals and families, and personality tests” (Hafez Training and Medical Center 2018).

Public discourse around psychiatry, as well as attitudes and expectations of the practice, are formed and maintained against the presumed dichotomy between psychodynamic and biomedical approaches. Although at the margins, psychoanalysis and the approaches arising from it remain influential, both among the public, as well as among the practitioners, the actual practice of such approaches remain scarce due to limitations on time and money. In Behrouzan’s words, psychiatrists in Iran practise in an ‘in-between’ space within psychiatry: “On the one hand, the medical establishment’s attitude toward psychoanalysis oscillates perplexingly between acknowledgement and rejection. On the

[1] Although the 5th revision of the DSM was published in 2013, and the translation into Farsi was completed in 2015, the criteria in use by practitioners in Iran continues to be DSM-IV-TR, at the time of completion of this study.

other hand, psychodynamic psychiatry, neither absent nor holding a deserved status, continues to inform Iranian psychiatry in creative ways" (Behrouzan 2016, p. 207). It is within such pedagogical and professional understanding and the way they inform broader pre-defined cultural norms and conceptualisations, that individuals in Iran understand mental disorders, and make sense of their own experiences of these illnesses.

Sadness, Dysphoria, and Conception of Life in Iran

Literature on depression in Iran is scarce. However, medical anthropologists Byron Good and Mary-Jo Good conducted one of the few studies on the topic in 1970s. A central conclusion they draw from their observations in Iran, one that merits a closer look, is that sadness and dysphoria are valued emotions in Iranian culture, and even encouraged: "Dysphoria – sadness, grief, despair – is central to the Iranian ethos, an emotion charged with symbolic meaning" (Good et al. 1985, p. 384). This claim defines a cultural framework for understanding depression in Iran, since it presents a case where the boundaries between what is considered normal and pathological are blurred. The centrality of sadness and dysphoria in Iran is based on observations of cultural and religious rituals, as well as works of literature. Good and Good argue that the importance of dysphoric affects and experiences pertaining to them, as seen in Iranian culture, find meaning within two frameworks; "one associated with an understanding of the person or self, the other with a deep Iranian vision of the tragic", as expressed in various cultural mediums and interpretations (Good et al. 1985, p. 385).

Whilst I agree that various cultural rituals and mediums are concerned with some form of dysphoric affect, I disagree that the presence of sadness in these occasions is a sign of the positive cultural valuation of this affect. The importance of sadness and dysphoric affect should rather be seen as a consequence of the cultural conceptualisation of life. Granted that the status of such emotions has notable implications for the conceptualisations and experiences of depression in Iran, it is important to understand the significance and place of these emotions within the cultural context. Taking the aforementioned pillars of the cultural context of Iran, it can be shown that despite having a special place in the religion, literature and interpretations of history, sadness and dysphoria are not valued for their own sake. Furthermore, the emphasis placed on these emotions is revealing of a fundamental cultural conceptualisation of life among Iranians that also plays a role in conceptualisations and experiences of depression.

Shi'ism

Good et al. observe that "the core of Iranian Shi'ism embodies a vision of the tragic and of grief as a religiously motivated emotion" (Good et al. 1985, p. 387). This claim is rooted in observations of the religious ceremonies and rituals, which take place on a regular basis in Iran.[2] Although some of these events are joyful and celebratory (e.g. Mid-Sha'ban, Mab'as, Eid al-Fitr), the majority (and the most important) of the ceremonies and rituals are aimed at commemorating the lost lives of religious figures and are thus centred around feelings of loss, grief and sadness. The latter group of religious occasions make up the main part of public religious ceremonies seen in Iran, with a considerable public participation. Based on the observation of these events, Kleinman and Good note, "For Shi'ite Muslims in Iran, grief is a religious experience, associated with recognition of the tragic consequences of living justly in an unjust world; the ability to experience dysphoria fully is thus a marker of depth of person and understanding" (Kleinman and Good 1985, p. 3). It is important to emphasise that the grieving and sadness associated with these events is not limited to that of the loss of a person, religious or otherwise. Rather, the lives and individuals commemorated symbolise the broader cultural ideal, namely the sacrifices made by the forces of Good, in the fight between Good and Evil.

The most important of the rituals for Shi'ite Iranians is one commemorating the death of the third Imam of Shi'ite Muslims, Hussein,

---

[2] It should be acknowledged that most of these events are supported by the state, ensuring the regularity of the events, as well as the wide reach of them around the country.

whose tale of life and death symbolises bravery and fighting for justice in a world of injustice (Fischer 1980). On the day of Ashura, Hussein and his army of 72 fought against an army of thousands in the Battle of Karbala and the war ended with the death of Hussein and all of his men. In the rituals commemorating these events, the tale of the battle of Karbala is told and retold through different mediums such as public performances (*ta'zieh*) or mourning ceremonies (*hey'at-e azādāri*). Hundreds of people attend these ceremonies, to hear the tale of the battle and the sacrifices made by Imam Hussein and his followers, while weeping, beating their chests and grieving. Despite the differences in form and shape, the common factor linking all of these ceremonies together is the public display of sorrow with large groups of people participating in them. It is this factor, whose observation leads researchers to conclude that such religious ceremonies are a public manifestation of a personally felt sadness, one that is static in nature and thus ready to be publicly expressed routinely.

Despite appearances, what is more fundamental than the public display of sadness and sorrow in this and other similar events, is the emphasis placed on the fight between the forces of Good and Evil. What is relived in the ceremony of Ashura, is the remembrance of the bravery and the values held by the Imam and his willingness to die for these values. The battle of Karbala is the ultimate representation of what Iranians take to be the very essence of life itself, i.e. a fight between the forces of Good and Evil. And Hossein, as one of the most adhered to role models for Shi'ite Iranians, represents the good person fighting this fight, suffering inevitable pain in his efforts to be on the side of good, battling evils of injustice, unfairness, and cruelty. Viewed in this way, the annual ceremonies commemorating this battle act as reminders of the injustices and evil that exist in this world, and of the fact that being good is inevitably accompanied by pain and suffering and sadness. Understood as such, it is not the case that the religious ceremonies and rituals provide a platform for the display of sadness. Rather, sadness is construed as the necessary consequence of being on the side of Good, in the eternal fight between Good and Evil.

The notion of Good and Evil is emphasised in various religious texts and teachings, and thus is part of the religious culture of Iran. However, this understanding is not limited to the religious domain, and rather is part of the broader cultural conceptualisation of life, which can be found in Iranian culture long before it endorsed Islam.

Persian Poetry and Literature

Good et al. view the exploration of dysphoric affects in works of literature as another indicator of the centrality of sadness as a valued emotion in the Iranian culture. They specifically examine the modern secular literary works, as "they explicitly explore the boundary between pathology and a valued sense of tragic, exploring the meaning of despair, pathological grief, and suicide" (Good et al. 1985, p. 389). Although these themes are indeed present in the most influential works of Iranian literature in the twentieth century, similar themes of the tragic, grief, and loss have been present in Iranian works of literature throughout history, within the broader conception of life as a fight between Good and Evil. These themes can be found in the ancient religion of Zoroastrianism, especially in the Gathas—the hymns at the heart of the religion—, as well as in ancient Persian mythologies. It is from such starting points that the themes are seen in works of literature over the centuries.

An instance of where this cultural conceptualisation is seen in works of literature, is in *The Book of Kings (Shāhnāmeh)*, dubbed "the national epic of Persia" (Encyclopaedia Iranica 1999). Written by Ferdowsi around the tenth century, the work revisits ancient Persian mythologies, but with real mortal people in place of the forces and the ancient gods. The epic tells stories that are often concerned with tragedies of loss, grief, injustice and war, which find meaning in the eternal fight between forces of Good and Evil. The most well-known and influential story in the book is what is arguably the most sorrowful of all, telling the tale of a father and son, symbols of bravery and chivalry, who have to endure immense suffering. Sohrāb unknowingly enters a battle with his father, Rostam, and gets fatally wounded. After realising that he has wounded his own son, Rostam tries to find an antidote to heal Sohrāb, but the medicine arrives only after Sohrāb's death. Now Rostam, who is portrayed as incredibly strong and unbeatable, is filled with sorrow, guilt and grievance. The depiction of these feelings is a detailed and powerful account, comprising, similar to the religious tales, the themes of grievance and loss. And similar to the religious tales, these themes find meaning in a broader context of the fight between Good and Evil, where a person who is a symbol of bravery and strength, falls victim to a conspiracy of a few thirsty for power. It is within this broader theme that the truth is kept from Rostam, and he is made to endure the guilt of killing his own son, and the grief of his loss.

The theme of the war between the forces of justice and injustice and the resulting sacrifices is also seen in *The Book of Kings* in the story of the death of Siāvash. He is one of the most innocent characters in the epic, who falls victim to the jealousy of others. Despite proving his innocence over and over again, Siāvash becomes the victim of an elaborate plot that results in his painful unjust death. He, who believed in his innocence and was filled with love, refused to fight, and the other side, deceived by the jealousy of its people, took him away and brutally took his life. The account following his death is not only concerned with the state of the world that has taken the life of an innocent man, but also the shame and guilt and grievance felt by the deceived side upon knowing the truth. The emphasis put on righteousness and innocence, together with the appraisal of truth and condemn of jealousy, makes clear certain parallels with the religious ceremonies. The aim of retelling the stories, whether of the fictional battles in the *The Book of Kings*, or those of the religious figures is one and the same: the commemoration of forces of good. The sadness and the sorrow at the centre of these tails, come from seeing and appreciating the suppression of these forces of good.

Themes of sadness and dysphoria found in the more recent works of literature, also find their meaning within this broader conception, albeit they approach the matter from a different perspective. Good et al. look at the example of a twentieth century novel, *The Blind Owl* by Sadegh Hedāyat, which explores themes of sadness and melancholy from a social perspective. Here, the concern is with the fight of an individual for authenticity, in the face of a society that limits him, causing him suffering and despair. The concern here is the same as the early works of literature, and the religious ceremonies. Life itself is construed as a fight between Good and Evil, manifested in different forms—unjust war, struggle of individual vs the society, etc.—, with those on the side of Good facing inevitable sadness and suffering.

Iran in the 1980s

Another domain where the emphasis on sadness and dysphoria can be seen in the Iranian culture, is in the interpretations of historical events. This is seen in the commemorations of Hussein as centred around a particular reading of historical events. Yet a more revealing example is the Iran-Iraq war and understanding of the events against the backdrop of cultural conceptions, where similar themes as those in the works of literature and religious ceremonies, are revisited. During the war, the length of battles was justified by appealing to the fight between the forces of Good and Evil, with the Iranian side unquestioningly on the side of the Good. The official discourse after the war, continues to make this association, aiming to keep the memories of war alive, whilst sanctifying its horrors. For instance, the tales of those killed in the war were made into compulsory school curricula—most famously the story of Hossein Fahmideh, a 13-year-old who was killed at the beginning of the war. Giant murals of those killed were put up on streets and highways (and remain until the present day), and roads and alleys everywhere are named after them. Within the dominant discourse, the confrontation with Iraq has never been a 'war', but 'The Holy Defence', and those killed are not 'casualties' but 'martyrs'.

Various national ceremonies commemorating the sacrifices of war and the lives lost, emphasise the same themes as those visited in the religious ceremonies, namely the eternal fight between Good and Evil. It is true that Iran suffered heavy losses and destruction, but these are justifiable since Iran was the one fighting on the side of Good, and as such, the loss and suffering was not only inevitable, but remains something to be proud of. By keeping the memories of war alive, therefore, the public is reminded, not only that there is an eternal fight between forces of Good and Evil, but also that being on the side of Good brings with it inevitable pain, suffering and sadness. Thus, by encouraging people to be on the side of Good, the inevitability and the desirability of suffering as a sign of moral superiority is emphasised.

The significance of this analysis is twofold. First, it refutes the claim that sadness and dysphoric affect are valued in the Iranian culture. It is a mistake to take public displays of sadness, and the emphasis on these emotions in other domains of Iranian life, as a positive valuation and encouragement towards such feelings for their own sake. Rather, this emphasis finds meaning against broader cultural modes of understanding and interpretation. The inevitable sadness that one endures by attempting to be good, is seen as meaningful and significant. It is valued because it signals the individual's good intentions and pure heart. And it is the fact that this kind of sadness is meaningful that distinguishes it from what is to be considered as abnormal, meaningless, and pathological.

#41(F) – Depression is very different [to sadness and sorrow]. Other forms of sadness have a clear reason, but in depression one gets confused and loses the reason.

#39(F) – Depression is very different [to sadness and sorrow], it brings seclusion/isolation and you are sorrowful all by yourself. But one can tolerate sadness and sorrow, and can leave it to God.

Secondly, the analysis highlights the cultural conception of life as an ongoing, and never-ending fight between the forces of Good and Evil. This cultural conception is noteworthy as a powerful cultural framework, against which various experiences find meaning and are made sense of. Furthermore, the observation that as a broad cultural conceptualisation instances of this understanding can be seen in different forms and in different domains of life, highlights the importance of acknowledging this conceptualisation in a study concerned with Iranian cultural frames of thought and understanding. Indeed, in exploring the influence of culture on experiences of depression, the understanding of life as a fight between Good and Evil, can be shown to be a recurring and important cultural influence.

Conceptualisation of Depression in Iran

The place of sadness and dysphoric affect in Iranian culture, and the respondents' clear distinction between these emotions and depression, raises the question as to how depression is understood in the Iranian culture and the various elements affecting this conceptualisation. This is an important question to answer at the outset, since in the case of psychiatric disorders both the diagnosis and the characteristics are known through means which, rather than being universal and empirically determinable, are often influenced by personal, sociological, and cultural factors. In diagnosing depression, for instance, the primary indicators come from personal reports of experiences that are thought to be abnormal and debilitating. Here, the personal articulations come about and find meaning within a broader sociocultural framework for thought and interpretation, as do the judgments of what constitutes an abnormal experience or behaviour. Understanding psychiatric disorders as diseases, ones that remain universal and empirically observable, despite cultural variations that only superficially muddy the picture, thus making the observation of the universal characteristics more difficult, does not give an accurate picture of mental disorders. More importantly, such a characterisation of mental disorders would be unhelpful for the purposes of cross-cultural study of depression. Rather, the role of culture, as a system of understanding and interpreting mental disorders must be acknowledged, *even if* there is a biological underlying cause of experiences of mental illnesses. This recognition demands a preliminary account of cultural conceptualisations of depression, through which individuals make sense of their experiences of depression. Behrouzan (2016) has offered an extensive account of how shared historical experiences and generational memories, form the basis of understanding *depreshen* for a generation of Iranians who grew up during the war. There are, however, other broader cultural modes of thought and understanding that also carry significance in understanding, and encountering depression in Iran today.

Traditional Iranian and Islamic Medicine

Although mental illnesses have been a subject of discussion in traditional medicine, the broader influence of this field has been on the cultural conceptualisation of health and illness, as well as ways of preventing and treating ill health. Iranian traditional medicine, especially as developed in the Islamic era (from the seventh century onwards), has remained influential throughout the years among Iranians. There has also been a renewed interest in the subject in the recent years in Iran, with the creation of a Traditional Medicine department within Tehran University of Medical Sciences, dedicated to teaching and research. The continued influence of traditional medicine shows that it forms part of the cultural way of understanding health and illness, and individuals' methods for encountering different illnesses.

In the understanding of traditional medicine, the physiological functions of the human body are based on factors such as elements, temperaments, humors, and forces (Rezaeizadeh et al. 2009). Traditional Iranian medicine gives more attention, and attaches more importance to the prevention of disease, rather than curing it, thus the primary role of a physician is to keep people healthy, and secondarily to cure them if sickness arises. Good health is understood as a state of balance between various elements in the human body, such as the humors, and those in the individuals' environment, such as 'good air', lack of stressors and cleanliness of the environment. So long as this balance is maintained, individuals enjoy a state of health, whilst the disruption of this balance gives rise to ill health and disease. Within this understanding, therefore, diseases are understood as natural events, and as such can be alleviated using natural means which could restore the balance in the body. Such natural treatments often include a change in habits, such as one's diet, and the use of medicinal plants and herbal remedies.

Interestingly, although in this understanding disease is essentially a physical phenomenon, a healthy mind is also seen as essential in maintaining a general state of health. This is since in traditional Iranian medicine there is no strict separation between mind and body, and rather, the two are seen as interdependent, and influencing one another. As such, stress factors such as worry, anxiety and unhappiness are seen as states of ill-health of the mind, which can threaten the healthy state of the body. Stress is further seen as an important factor, through which many physical symptoms and sicknesses, such as headache, back pain, fatigue, and blood pressure, can be accounted for and treated. With such importance, various stressors in life are identified as the ultimate 'causes' of disease. These stressors can be due to pressures from the environment such as work, relationships or studies, as well as from more abstract sources such as jealousy or The Evil Eye (Loeffler 2007). It is acknowledged that stress cannot be avoided altogether in life, and therefore one should aim to deal with stress in such a way as to maintain one's state of health. It is believed, therefore, that the drugs prescribed for diseases caused by stressors merely treat the symptoms and leave the root cause of the illness intact. Thus, "dealing with stress, learning to cope with it or avoiding it altogether, is considered to be a more satisfactory and desirable treatment than pharmaceutical remedies allopathic doctors recommend" (Loeffler 2007, p.56).

Within this conceptualisation, although the environment is a key element in the understanding of health and disease, these latter are ultimately understood in physical terms. The emphasis on the body and maintaining a humoral balance is such that psychological states, such as emotions, can also be understood in physiological terms. For instance, "anger is the boiling of the blood in the heart and the movement of the natural heat, which is sent outward to the rest of the body; it can be seen by redness in the eyes and a flushed face" (Dols 1992, p. 64). Such a characterisation is important because by giving a physiological account of how emotions come about, traditional medicine defines a close relation between physical and psychological states. Such a relation, in turn, can be used in treating diseases, of psychological and emotional nature, as well as those primarily affecting the body. Within this understanding "emotional states were, thus, able to influence directly the qualities in the body. Like food or drink, emotional states, such as happiness or anger, could be induced in a patient to counteract a humoral imbalance or physical condition" (Dols 1992, p. 159). The conviction that psychological and emotional states can also be understood in physical terms, implies that purely mental diseases, if in existence, are incurable, since treatment is only a viable option for diseases of the physical body, which can be observed and examined. For instance, Ibn-Sina claimed that "people who imagine they can cure effeminate homosexuals are singularly stupid. For this is a mental –not a physical– disease" (Dols 1992, p. 97).

The continuous prevalence of this understanding of health and illness has an undeniable effect in shaping experiences of depression in Iran. This influence is not limited to how Iranians understand depression and their experiences of it but is also seen in the social understanding and judgments towards depression and those suffering from it (Chap. 5), as well as in the experience of somatic symptoms and the embodied experience of depression (Chap. 7).

Iranian Ideal Character Types

The second important element in shaping Iranian conceptions of depression and modes of encountering it, is what is considered to be an ideal kind of person in Iranian culture. Although there are gendered differences in such an ideal, informed by the sociocultural norms and expectations of men and women, some ideal characteristics apply to both men and women. The concern here is in the large part with values that are thought to be essential for a good person, regardless of their gender. This aspect also plays a role in shaping interpersonal relationships, social judgements of depression, and the resulting behaviours and attitudes in individuals (Chaps. 5 and 6).

There are two extremes in the stereotypical character traits among Iranians (Bateson et al. 1977). On the one hand, there are the negative traits often attributed to those in power when criticising the state of the society. These traits portray an image of an individual as calculating, opportunistic, and insincere. Such a characterisation attaches to the individual as a central characteristic, "a hidden purpose, a discontinuity between behaviour and intention" (Bateson et al. 1977, p. 262). In contrast with these traits, there are certain qualities that Iranians value in themselves and in their intimate circle of friends and family. In this category, traits such as honesty, kindness, modesty, sensitivity and being emotionally responsive are among the most mentioned. Given the influence of religious teachings, and especially Shi'ism, in Iranian culture, these positive traits are often attributed to religious figures and in particular to Ali, the first Imam of Shi'ite Muslims: "Hazrat-i Ali is the perfect man, and all virtues are ascribed to him" (Bateson et al. 1977, p. 263). Although there are various role models in Shi'ism, both male and female, who are adhered to,[3] Ali stands out as one of the most powerful

[3] Examples of such female role models include Fatemeh, the Prophet's daughter and Imam Ali's wife, whose purity of character, innocence, power to stand up to injustice, and support and care for her family are among her most celebrated personal characteristics.

of these, due to his positioning in Shi'ite Islam—as the first Imam hand-picked by the Prophet. In addition, a relatively large body of his written work has been preserved. These written letters and sermons, together with oral stories about him, detail not only his thoughts and ways of governing, but also his morale and conduct which make him a role model for a large part of Shi'ite Iranians.

At the heart of the specific traits attributed to Ali, is a sense of purity of the heart and integrity, termed *safā-yi bātin*. It is this characteristic that can be found at the centre of the positive valuations of an individual's character, and what individuals would aspire to. Literally translated as 'inner peace' or 'inner tranquillity', *safā-yi bātin* has embedded within it an important distinction made by Iranians in judging one's personality and character; between the interior and exterior of one's behaviour, what one appears to be and how one actually is inside. This dichotomy is seen in different terms and in different judgments of individuals, rooted in the religious teachings that preach good intentions (*niyyat-i khayr*), a good character (*sīrat*) as well as a good face (*sūrat*). In this characterisation, negative judgments and criticism towards individuals often take the form of an attack on their character, for failing to have purity of heart, thereby causing and manifesting a discontinuity between intention and behaviour. As such, *safā-yi bātin* functions both as an aspect of many Iranians' self-image, or a trait they aspire to, as well as being the characteristic expected to guide personal relationships.

Purity of heart, or *safā-yi bātin*, therefore, can be thought of as the most important marker of what Iranians consider to be a good person, and the ideal character type to aspire to. It should be noted that the person identified with *safā-yi bātin* carries certain other desirable qualities as well. For example, such a person has a certain depth of character, is self-reflective, and is aware of the goings-on around her. This characteristic is associated with religious figures such as Ali, and therefore there is often the expectation that a person with this attribute would also be a devout Shi'ite. However, increasingly this association and the resultant religious expectations are replaced with general non-religious moral standards. What does remain, is the association of such a person with other morally superior characteristics, seen both in Islamic teachings and in broader

Iranian conceptualisations. Notably, such a person, with her depth of character, honesty and appreciation of the ongoing fight between Good and Evil that constitutes life, and with her inner peace and purity, seeks to be 'good' in the spiritual and immaterial way that is celebrated in religious figures.

Understanding this cultural way of evaluating one's character and personality is important for the discussion at hand for two main reasons. First is the association of the valued characteristics with religious figures, which signals the cultural tendency of measuring oneself up against these figures. As will be seen later on, the adherence to these individuals makes the case for their teachings forming part of the cultural consciousness. As such, their teachings have a role to play in understanding part of the cultural sources of variation in experiences of depression and their articulations. Secondly, these cultural modes of evaluation play an important role in social and interpersonal relationships and the way these are disrupted in depression. As I will show, the dynamics of the breakdown of interpersonal bonds can in part be analysed with reference to such modes of evaluation and judgements of character.

Causal Attributions in the Cultural Context

It is noted in the psychological literature that members of collectivist societies are more likely to attribute the cause of events in their lives, especially the negative ones, to an outside source (e.g. Choi et al. 1999; Carpenter 2000; Triandis 2002). This externalising approach is in part due the conception of self in these societies as dependent on the collective group, which has consequences for ascribing responsibility for a certain action or event. Iran, as a collectivist culture and society, is not an exception to this idea. This characteristic in Iran, however, goes beyond the individual persons' ideas of causes of events in their lives, and has been discussed in theories about the broader Iranian identity and culture.

Among Iranian modern intellectuals who attempt to analyse and understand historical events and their consequences, almost always the causes of misfortune and lack of success have been attributed to external forces of influence; whether through waging war, or more insidious forces of Imperialism. The few intellectuals who have not followed this trend, stand out as especial cases, such as the writer and thinker Sadegh Hedayat (e.g. Hedayat 2002).

Despite their influence, it would be a mistake to see these conceptions as unique to intellectuals. They have rather formed part of the dominant discourse among public figures, including politicians and policy makers, and, more importantly, the general public. For instance, in popular culture, the supposed decline of the Iranian nation as a whole is often attributed to the Arab invasion of the seventh century, and later to the influence of 'the English' (as seen in the immortalised novel of Iraj Pezekshzad, *My Uncle Napoleon* (2006/1963)). This cultural way of encountering 'the Other' and the almost instinctive and automatic attempt to guard oneself against it, arguably has its roots in ancient, pre-Zoroastrian worldview, where the distinction between Self and Other is between *Iran* and *aniran* (non-Iranian). This differentiation has carried over through history and been maintained in the dominant belief system of the country:

> In Zoroastrian texts, and with a remarkable resonance later in Shi'i Islam, such differentiation carried important political implications. In the cosmic struggle between forces of the good supporting Ahuramazda (the God of Wisdom) and forces of evil supporting Ahriman, the Iranians are naturally perceived as being on the side of the good. That meant that they had to be constantly on guard against impurities and evil pollutants that originate from the aniran. If left unchallenged, these alien forces were to prevail either by violent means or through deception, that would corrupt the believers' communal and individual bodies. (Amanat 2012, p. 11)

This brief exposition serves to show that the causal attribution of an event, especially a negative one, to a source outside of oneself, whether an individual self or as part of a bigger national self-identity, is not merely the result of the collectivist nature of the society but is a more general cultural tendency. Furthermore, certain parallels can be drawn between this conceptualisation and the ideal character types noted previously, where the suspicion of a powerful Other not only guides one's encounters with others, but also forms the basis for distinguishing one's inner peace and purity of the heart from the Other's dishonest hidden intentions.

Conceptualisations of Depression in Questionnaire Responses

The three elements explored here as influencing the Iranian conceptions of depression, are indeed reflected in the responses to the questionnaire, particularly in how respondents define depression, and what they see as having caused their depression. In instances respondents view depression as an 'illness of the soul', or a state of 'imbalance' in the soul, since depression is rarely associated with physical symptoms, and is seen as distinct from physical illnesses.[4]

#1(F) – When the state of one's soul (*hāl-e roohi-e ādam*) becomes unbalanced and goes towards a continuous (*mostamar*) sadness (*ghamgin shodan*), it is depression.
#19(F) – Depression is illness of soul and spirit.
#22(F) – Depression is an illness of the soul and problems in life caused me to become depressed.

Alternatively, there are those who, in line with the conceptualisation of health and illness in traditional medicine, view depression as rooted in physical disturbances that influence one's mind.

#2(M) – [Depression is] a physical process that happens in the body and ends in depression or as some might say, problems of the soul.
#21(F) – [Depression is caused by] diet and [genetic] inheritance—my mother has depression.

A significant number of respondents identify external causes for their depression, among them environmental stressors that are hinted at in traditional medicine conceptualisations. There are also cases where other people, their bad behaviour and/or intentions are seen as bringing about depression, highlighting the idea of one's inner purity being tainted by external forces.

[4] This is despite the prevalence of complaints of somatic symptoms among the Iranian sample. I will look at these symptoms more closely in Chap. 7.

#16(F) – In the process of getting divorced and when I was engaged I endured difficult circumstances and that caused my depression.
#17(F) – I became depressed after failing the Konkour [national university entrance exam] and the death of my fiancé.
#20(F) – Death of the dear ones has caused my depression, the pitying and humiliation because of this sadness has caused it. That I used to go to the cemetery and cry, and that others humiliated me for this caused my depression.
#33(M) – Depression [is], unsuccessfulness, being suppressed financially and physically, emotional incidents, and lacking a support network. Not having a job or an investment, not having social insurance, losing the dear ones [has caused my depression].
#37(F) – [Depression is] Not believing in oneself, having stress, of course in occasions which are not really under anyone's control.
#42(M) – Depression is a mental pressure, which is injected into one as a result of problems in life.

Chapter Summary

The themes explored in this chapter provide the context for the discussions and analyses in the later sections. As I will show, each of the themes touched upon here, present important elements against which the experiences and debates around depression as seen in Iran find meaning. The demographic make-up of Iran has important consequences for the attitudes and frames of reference that different social and age groups have in understanding depression. Cultural elements such as traditional medicine, ideal character types, and cultural modes of causal attributions have shaped the Iranian conceptions of depression, while the changing emphasis on the approach to psychiatry and public discourse, has influenced Iranians' understanding of psychiatry and their expectations of practitioners and different treatments. Whilst the different cultural, religious, and historical elements have led to various ways of defining and understanding depression, the interrelation of these elements is played out in the way depression is experienced and made sense of in the culture. The conceptualisation of life as an ongoing and eternal fight between the forces of Good and Evil, and the perception and aspiration of oneself being on the side of Good, has tangible influences on the way in which Iranians understand and interpret various aspects of their experience of depression. This conceptualisation, furthermore, underlies the distinctions Iranians make between the normal sadness and suffering that is seen as an inevitable part of being Good, and the pathological feelings experienced in depression. With this framework for meaning making and understanding in mind, and making use of the different elements detailed here, in the following chapters I will attempt to make sense of the Iranian experiences of depression and how they compare to those seen in the UK.

3

Metaphors of Depression

Metaphors are central in the way we think of ourselves, our experiences, and the world we live in. They are "pervasive in everyday life", not just because they provide us with a tool to talk about abstract ideas, or to convey feelings and emotions that are difficult to communicate in ordinary language, but also because "our ordinary conceptual system, in terms of which we both think and act, is fundamentally metaphorical in nature" (Lakoff and Johnson 1980, p. 3). Metaphors can be informative about the cognitive structures of our minds and modes of thinking, as well as the culture-specific domains of knowledge and belief against which the metaphors sometimes find meaning. A shared history can lie at the heart of the formation and use of a metaphor across cultures, while different cultural, physical, and environmental experiences can give rise to metaphors unique to the context in which they are used.

The role of metaphors in constructing and communicating narratives of illness experience have been well-documented (Sontag 1983; Sontag 1990; Charon 2006). The important role of metaphoric language is also visible in the domain of mental illness, for these can be so alien and unfamiliar that ordinary language would fall short of providing an accurate description of them. As an illness situated at the intersection of physical, emotional, and cognitive realities, and carrying symptoms

M. Mirdamadi, *A Phenomenological Study of Depression in Iran*,
https://doi.org/10.1007/978-3-031-30407-1_3

within each of these domains, depression gives rise to complex experiences. The complexity of these experiences often has consequences for the narratives of depression; the way we understand and know it, and the way those suffering from depression attempt to describe and explain their experiences. The definition of depression does not follow a universal and straightforward equation-like format, one that is easily understood, and has universal implications for any individual experiencing it. In the absence of such straightforward definitions, and "[w]hen equations fail, metaphoric and figurative language often provide an alternative mode of explanation" (Emmons 2010, p. 94).

Noting this importance, the concern in this chapter is to examine the universal, as well as culturally specific metaphors of depression. Given the way in which cultural scripts and ideas permeate our language and narratives of experiences, looking at common metaphors used across different cultures offers an insight into different elements of experiences of depression. Understanding the use of metaphors can illuminate, for example, the perceived nature of depression (e.g. a scary intruder as seen in characterisations of depression such as 'The Beast' by Tracy Thompson (1996)), and the change in one's perception of the world, brought about by depression (e.g. as falling in 'darkness' or the world 'losing its colour'). This analysis demonstrates that while some metaphorical narratives of depression describe the universal underlying experiences of depression, understanding of others requires situating the narrative and the individual experiences within a specific cultural context. This begs the question as to the relationship between variations in metaphors and in experiences: what does the variation in metaphors tell us about depression itself, as experienced across cultures? Does the variation in metaphors used in description amount to differences in how depression is experienced across cultures?

Cognitive-Linguistic Framework and Universal Metaphors for Depression

If we accept the universality of depression as an illness category, we would expect at least some of the experiences and understandings of the disorder to be universal. This universality would also extend to narratives and metaphors used to communicate depression across cultures. Research suggests that there are indeed such metaphors; ones denoting what could be thought of as the universally identifiable experiences of depression. The cognitive-linguistic framework for metaphors, put forward by George Lakoff and Mark Johnson, offers a way of discerning the significance of universal metaphors and the way in which they highlight an underlying universal experience.

Metaphors enable us to communicate our subjective mental landscapes to others by way of mapping the more abstract conceptions to domains of tangible everyday experiences. We may, for instance talk of importance (an abstract notion) in terms of the air that we breathe (sensorimotor experience in the world); or describe love and affection (subjective emotional experiences) in terms of warmth (a familiar physical sensation). Similarly, we conceptualise the understanding of an idea, as a subjective experience that is construed in abstract terms, in terms of grasping an object, which is based in our sensorimotor experience in the physical world and talk of 'grasping an idea'. The cognitive-linguistic framework explains this mapping by arguing that "metaphors are based on embodied human experiences" (Kövecses 2005, p. 2), which are often traceable to our experiences in childhood.

Associations between our non-sensorimotor subjective experiences and sensory experiences are developed very early on, during the time when the two types of experiences are conflated. Although later on we do indeed differentiate between these two forms of experience, the associations built up during the conflation period remain with us and form the basis for *primary* metaphorical conceptualisations (Lakoff and Johnson 1999, p. 46). An example of this kind of conceptualisation is the primary metaphor AFFECTION IS WARMTH (small capital letters denote concepts rather than words). Understanding affection in terms of warmth, can naturally be understood in terms of our embodied experiences and the conflation of the physical sensation of warmth with the emotional experience of affection. This correlation of the two experiences means that the two are undistinguished from one another during the period of conflation, when associations between affection and warmth are built up. These associations remain in place in our minds even after the experiences are differentiated and form the basis of the way we conceptualise affection, leading us to speak of '*warm* smiles' or 'having a *warm* relationship'. Primary metaphors formed in this way, it is argued, are most often universal in their use, since they arise as a result of universal experiences. Although it is conceivable that these metaphors do not appear in each and every culture, their use is widespread enough for them to classify as universal metaphors.

Primary metaphors, with their minimal structure, arise "naturally, automatically, and unconsciously through everyday experience by means of conflation, during which cross-domain associations are formed" (Lakoff and Johnson 1999, p. 46). The construction of primary metaphors in this way is aided by the neural activities in the brain, for the associations arise via "neurally instantiated correlation" between the sensorimotor and subjective experiences, so that the conflation of the two is the result of "simultaneous activation of the respective neural network" (ibid., pp. 54–55). As such, the neural connections established in the period of conflation 'project' inferences "from the sensorimotor *source network* to the subjective judgment *target network*" (ibid., p. 55), thus forming the basis for the mapping of primary metaphors. It is through this network of cognitive and neural learning that the conflations of domains of experience form the basis for the future learning and developing of primary conceptual metaphors. This is since, in the differentiation stage, domains of experience that were previously seen as concurrent and correlated "are differentiated into metaphorical sources and targets" (ibid., p. 49).

Primary metaphors are significant in this framework since, in addition to offering a way for placing metaphors within our conceptual framework, they also form the constitutive parts of more complex metaphors, which form a large part of our conceptual system, affecting the way we think and what we care about. These complex metaphors, in turn, and due to their pervasiveness in our thoughts, form the basis for further metaphorical combinations, both ordinary ones used in our everyday language, as well as poetic ones (Lakoff and Turner 1989). Primary metaphors combine to form complex metaphors through the mechanism of conceptual blending—that is, through inferences that make connections across different conceptual domains. As such, conceptual blending works by way of "the fitting together of small metaphorical 'pieces' into larger wholes" (ibid.). Primary metaphors therefore can be thought of atomic constitutive parts that create a larger molecular structure. Importantly, the way in which primary metaphors 'fit together' to make complex metaphors is, to some extent, dependent on the culture where they are constructed. This is since the cultural models and/or the folk theories and belief systems guide the structure of complex metaphors, ensuring that they reflect the widely-held beliefs and ideas in the culture where they are formed.

An example of a complex metaphor constructed in this way in the American culture, as noted by Lakoff and Johnson, is 'A PURPOSEFUL LIFE IS A JOURNEY'. This metaphor follows the folk model in the American culture, partly influenced by the teachings of the Bible, that people ought to have a purpose in life and to act so as to reach that purpose, while those who do not have one, are seen as 'lost' and 'without a direction in life'. This cultural model itself is made up of primary metaphors: PURPOSES ARE DESTINATIONS, and ACTIONS ARE MOTIONS, as can be seen by the metaphorical statement of the cultural belief that 'People ought to have destinations in life, and they ought to move as to reach those destinations'. The final element constituting the complex metaphor is the fact that a journey is made up of a long trip to a series of destinations. In this way, the metaphor A PURPOSEFUL LIFE IS A JOURNEY is seen to entail a complex metaphorical mapping from the abstract to the physical, including A PURPOSEFUL LIFE IS A JOURNEY, A PERSON LIVING A LIFE IS A TRAVELER, LIFE GOALS ARE DESTINATIONS, and A LIFE PLAN IS AN ITINERARY. (Lakoff and Johnson 1999, p. 61).

Applying this theoretical framework to the case of narratives of depression, McMullen and Conway (2002) have identified four conceptual metaphors for depression. With a sample size of over four hundred patients in the US, they examined patients' therapy sessions, reducing the often-varied wording and form of metaphors into basic conceptual metaphors using the cognitive-linguistic framework. These metaphors, in addition to tracing the historical development of conceptualising and understanding depression, can be traced to the physical experiences of depression, and as such are argued to be universal.

The first conceptual metaphor is DEPRESSION IS DARKNESS, which takes various forms, such as likening depression to a cloudy, rainy weather, as well as the patients describing themselves as feeling *dark* or being *blue.* As McCullen and Conway put it, "inherent in these phrases is … the sense of decreased clarity of consciousness and pervasively negative attitude and affect that are two of the hallmarks of depression" (McMullen and Conway 2002, p. 170). Additionally, these metaphors indicate the descent of depression upon the patient, seemingly autonomous and independent of the patient themselves. The second metaphor, often used to describe a sense of carrying a load around, is DEPRESSION IS WEIGHT. This metaphor is used to convey a sense of being weighted as felt in the whole body, rather than any particular part of it. McCullen and Conway see this as possibly amounting to not only a sense of being burdened, but also "of having one's freedom to move somewhat curtailed" (ibid., p. 171). Similar to this is the third metaphor DEPRESSION IS CAPTOR where patients communicate a sense of restriction, talk of feeling trapped by the illness and trying to break out and free themselves from it.

Despite the numerous variations of these metaphors, McCullen and Conway claim that these three metaphors only account for less than ten percent of all the metaphorical talk around depression, while the remaining ninety percent of instances of the use of metaphors is taken up by the most dominant metaphor: DEPRESSION IS DESCENT. This metaphor incorporates various expressions of being *low* or *down,* as the central descriptions of the patients' states, as well as "numerous metaphorical entailments or elaborations derived from our knowledge and experience of descent" such as the slow and difficult experience of pulling oneself up and out of an unwanted state or situation, after a quick and easy fall (ibid., pp. 171–172). As such, this conceptual metaphor fits in neatly within the framework advocated by Lakoff and Johnson in the sense that it conveys details of our knowledge and embodied experiences by means of mappings between the source domain and the target domain. These four metaphors also resonate with the embodied experience of depression, which will be looked at more closely in Chap. 7.

One way of looking at the widespread use of the metaphor DEPRESSION IS DESCENT, is thinking of it as a fundamental, basic metaphor of emotions, insofar as depression includes emotional changes and manifestations in the patient. Seen within the framework advocated by Lakoff and Johnson, the DEPRESSION IS DESCENT metaphor follows from the orientational metaphors of emotions. Lakoff and Johnson, as mentioned earlier, see primary metaphors as arising from our embodied experiences. In this sense, our primary metaphors for basic emotions, which are argued to be (largely) universal (Kövecses 2000, 2005; Lakoff and Johnson 1980), follow from our bodily sensations and posture when we experience them. For example, the primary metaphors of HAPPINESS IS UP, SADNESS IS DOWN have a physical bodily basis: "drooping posture typically goes along with sadness and depression, erect posture with a positive emotional state" (Lakoff and Johnson 1980, p. 15). DEPRESSION IS DESCENT follows directly from the place of such orientational metaphors in culture and incorporate within them the conceptualisation of depression as an undesirable, negative state, escaping from and 'pulling oneself out' of which requires immense effort and often proves difficult.

If the metaphor DEPRESSION IS DESCENT is indeed universal, then one would expect to find instances of it across different cultures. Indeed, in the case of depressed patients in Iran, there are various instances where people talk of 'falling into' depression, or trying to 'pull oneself out of' depressive states. In addition to indicating the embodied feeling of falling and being low, these metaphors also signify certain conceptualisations of depression as a dark pit or dungeon, which once one is fallen into, draws one in deeper. This sense of deep descent, together with the physical sensations like heaviness of the body, make the escape from this state ever more difficult. The presence of these metaphors in the Iranian sample further prove the case for the universality of this metaphor.

#18(M) – My depression world is like I have fallen into a dungeon (*siyāh-chāl*).

#13(M) – [When depressed] I want to sink into blackness even more.

FB#3 – … I am conscious that life in a city without sunshine, loneliness and being far from family and other personal elements have once again pushed me towards that black pit.

#10(F) – [Depression] is like a marsh that every moment sucks you in deeper.

Elements of the other three metaphors construed by McCullen and Conway as universal can also be seen in the above examples. Depression is viewed as a black and dark state which one falls into, and like a heavy weight pulls one in ever deeper. This way of understanding and describing depression further resembles the state of being captured by a force that does not allow for an easy escape. Although the metaphor of DEPRESSION IS DESCENT is more easily identifiable in the responses from the Iranian sample, some of the culture-specific metaphors used by the respondents also resemble the themes explored by McCullen and Conway, as I show in the following sections.

Culture-Specific Metaphors for Depression

Given the discussion so far, and the prominent theory for metaphors, the question remains as to how we ought to account for culturally variant metaphors. The cognitive-linguistic framework for metaphors, seems to leave little room for cultural variation in metaphors, since for the most part the account is concerned with universal experiences and biological elements that factor into the construction of metaphors. Recall that in this account, the role culture plays in the formation of metaphors is limited to complex metaphors. Specifically, it is argued that cultural modes of thinking guide the way in which primary metaphors fit together to form complex ones. But primary metaphors are formed as the result of experiences which are themselves largely universal, such as the experience of the infant being embraced by her parents. And as Lakoff and Johnson argue in their account, "universal early experiences lead to universal conflations, which then develop into universal (or widespread) conventional conceptual metaphors" (Lakoff and Johnson 1999, p. 46). If this were the case, one would expect to see that metaphors of depression across cultures are largely reducible to the few basic conceptual metaphors which are thought to be universal. In what follows, I will present two examples of prevalent metaphors used by depressed patients in Iran. As the analysis demonstrates, although some culturally specific metaphors can indeed be reduced to basic primary metaphors, this cannot be said for all of these. Instead, the understanding of such metaphorical communication and modes of narrative requires a deep understanding of the cultural concepts and frameworks for interpretation and understanding of experiences.

Talking in metaphors is customary in Iran, and it can be thought of as following from the long history of literature and poetry and their incorporation in everyday life and discourse of Iranians. One of the most widely used metaphors is that of colours, which gives a certain quality to a given situation. Such use of colour metaphors can be traced back to at least the twelfth century in the works of Rumi, where different colours are associated with different emotions, states of being and attitudes. For example, Rumi uses the colour red to signify, among other things, health and well-being, wealth and worth, and sometimes anger. Whereas green signifies life, nourishment and youthfulness, yellow is associated with shame, fear, and ailments. The colour black in these works is one often used to describe sadness, sorrow, mourning, and bitterness (Ansari et al. 2012). Such use of metaphors of colours continues to be commonplace both in contemporary literature, as well as in everyday discourse. It should also be noted that the metaphorical power of colours does not come solely from the association they have acquired in works of literature, rather, some colour terms are inherently metaphoric, in virtue of how they are named. The colour grey, for example, *khākestari*, literally means 'of or relating to ash'. The metaphorical uses of this colour term, in turn, can be interpreted in ways that go beyond the associated meaning as a colour term. Similarly, in other cases where the colours are named after different entities, such as water (colour blue) or different flowers (variations of purple and red), they take on the metaphorical meanings associated with those entities themselves, which are found in the works of literature, idioms, and everyday language.

As such, given the wide range of meanings associated with colour terms, it is not surprising that they have found their way into the everyday language of Iranians. In this context, metaphors of colour are most often used to positively state the existence of a certain mood or emotion as felt by the individual, or to convey a certain way in which the individual perceives the world. It is not uncommon, for example, for one to state that 'one's life has become black' (*roozegāram siyāh shod*) to state a disastrous state of one's being as a result of an event or a loss, or to wish someone to be happy and well by wishing them 'to be green' (*sabz bāshi!*). Given this outline of the place of colour metaphors in the Persian language, a look into the way these are employed by Iranians in describing their experiences of depression can be informative in understanding what may be considered the dominant mood of depression, as felt by Iranians.

As discussed in Chap. 2, previous studies on depression in Iran emphasise the importance of sadness and sorrow in the culture, and in experiences of depression (Good et al. 1985). Given these findings and the use of the colour term black in signifying emotions of sadness and dysphoria, one would expect to find different descriptions of depression making use of this metaphor. However, the use of this colour term, rather than representing a common theme, was limited to only a few instances.

#17(F) – The world seems black to me and I think it is not worthy at all. Every day is the same and repetitive … [the sadness] just becomes longer and like a black aura which takes over my whole being and entangles my whole life.
#13(M) – [I felt] the story of my life becoming black.

In contrast, the most frequent use of the concept of colour in people's articulations of their experiences of depression seems to be different to the common way of employing these terms. Whereas in everyday contexts colour terms are employed to state and describe an *existing* mood or emotion, in describing their experiences of depression, Iranians mostly talk of 'lack of colour', 'fading colours' or the world 'losing its colour'. Furthermore, the fact that such statements can be seen with regards to various aspects of life in depression, such as ways of seeing the world and one's relation to it, as well as effects of medication, I would argue that these statements give an account of the mood in depression generally, as it is felt by Iranians.

#1(F) – [When taking medications] sexual matters become colourless (*bi rang*) and even grotesque (*maskhare*).
#6(F) – [In depression] the positive aspects [of life] lose their colour (*kam rang*) and sometimes even vanish altogether.

#3(F) – […] in the end life is always a little bit interesting, but it can lose its colour (*kam rang*).
#10(F) – Life is vain (*bi-fāydeh*), colourless, tasteless and unreal.
#16(F) – [My relations with others] really faded in colour.

What is interesting here is the replacing of the usual use of colour terms as a descriptive tool and one that attaches certain qualities to different experiences and entities, with an image of the world with fading colours, or in some cases, a blank, colourless image where the existence of any attitude or feeling towards the world is uncertain. The metaphorical phrases used here are heavy in terms of the meaning they convey, as the images of a colourful vs. a colourless world are powerful in antithetical ways. A world full of colour is construed as one full of energy, representing emotionally meaningful possibilities and motivation to strive towards the future. In such an image the perception is one of a mobile world, where one can conceive of change, as opposed to being threatened by a mundane daily routine. This is while the colourless world is idle, and idly meaningless (the theme of meaninglessness will be explored further in Chap. 4). The atmosphere and mood in such a world is one of frustration, indifference and stillness. There is no motivation to move forward, since there is no perception of conceivable change. In such a world the only colour that could be seen is that of an enduring grey, if one counts grey as a colour at all.

#8(M) – [I feel] cold and grey.
FB#5 – [Depression] was grey (*khākestari*) … It was like a filter on my eyes. [Like] big grey eyeglasses that reveal a grey life.

These various elements of meaning embedded in these metaphors serve to give a good general picture of the mood in depression in Iran. This picture is further reinforced by the direct descriptions of inability to find meaning in life and everyday activities, by the lack of change, lack of hope, etc. What is further interesting, is the fact that sadness and sorrow are not emphasised as strongly as part of depression experience. Lack of colour and the colour grey, which signify neutrality and idleness, rather than sadness, are used considerably more in the responses in describing the mood in depression, compared to the colour black which is often used in everyday language to convey a sense of sadness and sorrow. It seems that one of the main constitutive parts of the experience of depression in Iran can be characterised through the perceived colourlessness of the world.

Depression is often portrayed in the UK and US with colours associated with sadness: black, and various shades of grey. Perhaps the most familiar example of such portrayal is the often-cited representation of depression as 'a black dog' which follows one everywhere (Johnston 2007). Or, as seen in the study conducted by McCullen and Conway, as the grey colour we associate with cloudy and rainy weather. Indeed, I would argue that the metaphors of colour themselves can be understood in terms of the conceptual universal metaphor THE WORLD IS COLOURFUL. This conceptual metaphor can further be traced to our physical experience in, and of the world. Due to our biological make up, and the physical properties of our visual system, people from different cultures, have access to the same colour palettes, and we all perceive the world as colourful. The cultural variation in these metaphors is seen in the association of different colours with different states and affects, leaving the universal conceptual metaphor intact. For example, whereas 'feeling blue' for English speakers means feeling sad or having a low mood, the colour blue in the Iranian culture, is often associated with the feeling of calmness and tranquillity. This is while the colour black in both cases is associated with a sense of sadness, loss, and sorrow. As such, both similarities and differences in the use of colour terms could be said to arise from the conceptual metaphor THE WORLD IS COLOURFUL.

In depression, however, the cognitive and emotional change that one goes through amounts to an altered perception of the world, which, despite some differences in representation across cultures, remains an integral part of the experience of depression. The perception of the world in depression as grey, in some sense amounts to the alteration of this perception of the world, changing our ordinary experience of the world as colourful into a colourless one. In this sense, the message conveyed by Iranians when they describe their various experiences and feelings of the world in depression as 'colourless', 'faded in colour' or 'losing colour' could indeed be equated with the message conveyed by patients in the US or UK, who talk of 'cloudy', 'rainy' and 'grey' world. This variation can also be due to certain geographical characteristics. The use of metaphors of rain and cloudy weather, in the US and UK, to signify the idleness of the world in depression can be traced to the abundance of such weather and the sense of familiarity and cultural associations with it which drive the metaphors. The absence of such metaphors in Iran can in turn be linked to its different climate where rain and cloudy weathers are less frequent, and therefore carry a different symbology in the culture and a weaker sense of familiarity. Despite the differences in the metaphors used to describe the prevailing mood in depression, the basic experience of depression that is conveyed in these different metaphors remains the same. In other words, the basic metaphor DEPRESSION IS COLOURLESSNESS can be extracted from both sets of patients. This metaphor arguably arises from the observation that there is a basic existential change (Ratcliffe 2008, 2015) in the way one perceives the world around her in depression, in ways that amount to feelings of idleness, lack of motivation and the struggle to find meaning, in a world that was previously seen as colourful and one that presented itself with various possibilities.

This way of accounting for the variation in metaphors across cultures, points to the fact that one's sensorimotor experiences can vary in accordance with the geographical and environmental context of the experiences. Such external variations, therefore, can give rise to various experiences that in turn give rise to variation in conceptual metaphors. As pointed out above, for example, the significance of rain in different geographical locations can give rise to different metaphors. In a country with a largely wet weather, rain can take on metaphorical meanings that capture the inconvenience of rain or the gloominess of a rainy weather. This is while in a different location where it rarely rains and the weather is largely dry, rain can come to symbolise happiness and fertility. A similar argument can be made for the dominant values in a society, which form the basis of cognitive conceptualisations of phenomena, which in turn give rise to conceptual metaphors. Thus, in a culture, such as Iran where sadness has a prominent place, metaphors of depression might aim to highlight other aspects of the illness such as the prevalent sense of meaninglessness and idleness (see Chap. 4), rather than the persistent sadness entailed in it. Such examples show that variation in metaphors across cultures, is not only found in complex metaphors which are formed in accordance with the cultural modes of thinking, but also in primary metaphors which are based in fundamentally different experiences brought about as a result of different cultural values, as well as environmental factors.

Indeed, there have been attempts within the cognitive-linguistic framework to modify the account in order for it to be more accommodating to cultural variation (e.g. Kövecses 2005). Kövecses argues that there is much more to be done for the cognitive-linguistic framework to become a comprehensive account of metaphors, one which could accommodate the universality of certain metaphors, as well as their cultural variations. Although Kövecses leaves the scope open for various sources of variation, he argues that these can be broadly attributed to two types of causes. On the one hand, variation in metaphors can arise due to differences in our experiences, while on the other hand, our metaphors vary due to the variation in cognitive styles and preferences we use in the creation of abstract thought. One of the advantages of defining these two broad classes of causes is the large scope it leaves for the influence of culture, since variation in both experiences and cognitive preferences can arise, at least partly, due to variation in culture. However, there might also be a disadvantage in having such a large scope for variation, since personal variations could leave us with a theory of metaphor that is person-dependent: where meaning of metaphors are to be found through intimate relation with the person using the metaphors, rather than having a pre-defined basis for interpretation. This, in fact, would cause further problems, since part of the assumption behind the use of metaphors, is the existence of a shared space of meaning between people of the same social group.

What is undeniable, is the fact that there are indeed different ways of constructing, interpreting, and using metaphors. I could take a reasonable guess at the meaning of a metaphor uttered in a language and a culture where I am not a native, as I could understand the experience or the rationale behind the construction of it. However, the fact remains that some metaphors are so deeply rooted in the language and culture of a people, that understanding their message would be near impossible without at least some inside knowledge of that culture. An example of such a metaphor, found in Iranians' descriptions of their experiences of depression, is that of water. This metaphor should be classed as a cultural, rather than a universal cognitive metaphor. The story of how this element came to occupy a central place in the Iranian domain of metaphors needs to be told in order to serve as a justification for classifying the metaphor in this way.

In ancient Persian mythologies, water was the symbol of life and was seen as a holy entity from which every material thing was created.[1] In the pre-Zoroastrian mythology, it is said that following the creation of the heavens, Hormozd (the ancient Persian God) created the Earth and all within it from water: "such is said, that the first creations were all from water, except for the people and the animals, since these are descended from the essence of fire" (Bahar 1997, p. 44—my translation). From the story of the creation of the world from water, we find the first symbology of water in the Persian texts, namely one associated with creation and birth.

The second mythological symbolising of water, which follows from the earlier one, is the association of water with second birth. This is since water is seen as "an archaic symbol of the womb and of fertility; also purification and rebirth" (Hall 1994, p. 111). This rebirth does not only correspond to a second life after death (as is found in ancient Egyptian mythology), it rather encompasses any form of psychological rebirth and is thus representative of change in one's life. This sort of symbology is best seen in the Persian epic stories rooted in ancient mythologies, namely the *Shāhnāmeh* (The Book of Kings). In many of the stories in this book, water presents the heroes with changes, in the form of newly found strengths, which later on allow them to achieve their goal and overcome the obstacles. As the prominent Iranian mythologist Bahar put it;

> Passing through water has a special importance in Iranian mythology. Most of the heroes pass through water before achieving an immense success. This is probably based on the belief that with each passing through water, a new birth occurs. Water is associated with a mother's womb and a new birth represents purity, holiness and new power. (Bahar 1997, p. 260—my translation)

[1] This symbology of course, is not unique to Ancient Persia and is in fact seen in mythologies of Ancient Egypt, Babylon, and India.

This idea is also found in Christianity and baptism, pointing to a common history of this symbology. But this shared history does not guarantee a shared metaphorical language with similar (if not the same) meanings.

Following from this symbolising of water, the third one is that of water as the source of immortality. In various stories from ancient Persian mythologies, as well as Islamic stories that appeared much later, one sees the notion of 'Water of Life' (*āb-e hayāt*), as one which many heroes and characters of the stories seek in order to gain immortality.[2] It is worth noting, however, that in these mythical stories, the heroes are never successful in gaining immortality, as if they chase only an imaginary notion, the Water of Life always slips from them. The only story in which the hero finds the Water of Life, found in the *Shāhnāmeh*, represents immortality as becoming one with the heavens, rather than living on Earth, among material things forever. This could in fact be traced to the earlier perceptions of water as holy and in a sense, with supernatural qualities.

The mythological and ancient symbols are important here, since they offer a way of understanding the development of the metaphorical language and symbology surrounding water, which persist today. It can be argued that the reason why symbology of water in Islam was readily accepted into the Iranian culture, was due to the existing conceptions of water as holy, and as the source of all life. In Islam too, water is seen as the origin from which all was created and the holiness of it is seen in the teachings which see water as a tool for cleansing dirt and impurities. Although such a symbolism dates back to Mithraism as practiced in the then Persia (circa sixth century BC), and is seen in the retelling of the mythological stories, such as the *Shāhnāmeh*, the place of this notion in today's Iran has been further established through the Islamic teachings, which also see water as purifying.

This purifying character of water is in large part only associated with flowing bodies of water, such as rivers, and this association has given rise to further modes of thinking about flowing and standing bodies of water.

---

[2] In the West, this notion can be seen in the Fountain of Youth, although the portrayal and the stories that follow are slightly different.

In Islamic jurisprudence (*fiqh*) only flowing bodies of water can be used to cleanse the impurities (*nejāsat*) and they keep this purifying character even if their volume is much less than standing bodies of water (Al-Najafi 1984). Flowing bodies of water, in addition to being seen as having a purifying quality, are also a symbol of change and mobility. The juxtaposition of the two ways of symbolising bodies of water, have led to various metaphorical expressions, in poetry as well as the everyday life, which sanctify flowing water, while conversely, the standing bodies of water symbolise the opposite. In this symbology, then, a stagnant body of water would soon lose its quality of life-giving and fertility and instead give rise to an undesirable and unworthy environment in which no hope of life and fertility could be found. This undesirable character arises from a lack of change and idleness of the water and represents a trap leading to nothingness and death. As such, whilst flowing water was seen as a symbol of life and fertility, stagnant and static bodies of water came to be known as symbols of idleness, worthlessness, and death.

The undesirability of stagnant bodies of water is also seen in the names given to such bodies. Most notably, for example is the compound name '*mordāb*', literally meaning 'dead water'. Although scientifically this word designates marshes, due to its inherently metaphorical name, in the everyday language it is used to signify stagnant bodies of water generally, which would include, in addition to marshes, swamps and ponds. Such a name, as seen also in the case of inherently metaphorical colour terms in Farsi, plays a significant role in the conceptualisation of stagnant bodies of water. The way *mordāb* is defined in the Farsi lexicon is also interesting, as the definition relies on the contrast between flowing and stagnant bodies of water: "mostly applied to non-flowing water, which is standing and unmoving, as opposed to water of river which has movement and way" (Dehkhoda 1962—my translation).

In the context of talking about their experiences of depression, Iranians make use of this extensive symbology of water, conveying various meanings traceable to the development of the place of water, as a symbol, in Iranian culture. Although the use of such metaphors has been limited in the questionnaire, the few existing ones are noteworthy in highlighting the place and meaning of such metaphors in Iran, as well as being informative of aspects of the Iranian conceptualisation and experiences of depression.

The first way in which Iranians use the metaphor of water to describe their state in depression, is seen in the likening of depression, to a stagnant body of water, in which they are trapped and cannot get out of.

#10(F) – It's like a *mordāb*, that every moment sucks you in deeper.

Such characterisation and understanding of depression as a *mordāb* is commonplace in publications and websites that aim to educate people on the topic. A phrase that can be found repeatedly in describing the experience of depression is 'floundering in the *mordāb* of depression' (*dast va pā zadan dar mordāb-e afsordegi*), to signify the struggle involved in the experience of depression and the attempts at overcoming the illness (e.g. Beytoote.com 2015). The simile is seen time and again in self-help publications as well: "There will be instances when your determination against unanswered questions and feelings of hopelessness will be challenged. But it is precisely in these moments that you must pull yourself out of the inner *mordāb* ever more forcefully" (Ghahremani 2014—my translation)

In addition to the use of *mordāb*, with the associations described earlier, it is worth noting here the parallels with the research done by McCullen and Conway in which the conceptual metaphor DEPRESSION IS DESCENT was found to be the most dominant metaphor for depression in the US. The quote from the Iranian sample and the common ways of thinking about depression in Iran, as noted above, serve as evidence for the universality of this way of conceptualising depression. Namely, as a state that makes the individual suffering from it descend to a lower place, whether it is one's low mood that makes one droopy, or the sense of drowning or getting sucked in. The above quote can therefore serve as an example of a complex conceptual metaphor, one which despite drawing on universal basic metaphors, is developed in a way as to reflect the cultural framework for thought and popular beliefs specific to the cultural context in which they are used. Such a metaphor, as seen earlier, arises from the embodied experiences of depression, part of which would be conceptualised by metaphors for basic emotions, but one that is formulated in culturally familiar terms, which conform to the established cultural beliefs, thoughts and conceptions of depression.

This metaphorical way of talking about depression is significant, as it says something about the perceived nature of depression among the Iranian patients. Following the associations of stagnant bodies of water, depression is seen not only as an undesirable state, but also as a dangerous trap, carrying notions of idleness and decay, posing as a destructive threat to the self. This portrayal to some extent resonates with the associations found in the use of colour metaphors, namely the view of depression as transforming one's life to an idle, unchanging state, but goes further in the characterisation of depression as not only undesirable but dangerous and deadly. Once one is fallen in such a trap, an overwhelming strength, stemming from the inner self or an external force, is needed in order to find a way out. It can therefore be argued that, although the basic conceptualisation of depression is the same as that found by McCullen and Conway, the story that is told about this conceptualisation, through this metaphor, is a uniquely cultural one, arising from deeply rooted cultural notions, symbols and associations.

There are also instances of metaphorical descriptions of experiences which are more difficult to place within the cognitive-linguistic framework and seem to be constructed following only the cultural associations and frameworks for thoughts. For instance, although the cultural associations around water view it as a cleansing and purifying entity, there is also the idea that if water itself becomes a source of impurity, then ridding oneself of pollutants could become impossible and unthinkable:

FB#21 – I realised that the soil of my being is too close to the sea of depression … just a little digging makes the foul water of depression come out, and as soon as your hand is dirtied with this water you are no longer scared of getting wet. Once your hand is dirtied with it, precisely like an irresistible addiction you keep digging and make that hole deeper … after a while you realise that there is nothing left of you, and you yourself have become a big hole that is now always full of water.

The metaphor of depression as a foul fluid that disturbs the inner purity of the individual, and with its insidious nature slowly takes over one's being, is consistent with understanding of depression in other cultures as an intruding entity that takes over one. However, the cultural symbology of water is also noteworthy here; that which is supposed to maintain and restore purity, itself becomes a source of impurity, and fills one up in a way that restoring the pure nature of oneself seems out of reach.

Although in this case the understanding is one of water filling one up and fundamentally changing the nature of one's being, the metaphor of water can also be used to talk about one's very nature. Talking of the self in depression as a rough and stormy body of water, as seen in the following example, represents another instance where the cultural use of metaphor does not correspond with the universal metaphorical ways of talking about depression:

#12(F) – I was like a puddle that kids had jumped into. Worried, messy, confused. Meditation didn't show me the future but calmed that water and created a self-confidence, that although I don't know who I am or what I will do but certainly nothing bad will happen to me.

The above quote can be thought to be representing feelings of anxiety that often accompany depressive symptoms. What is interesting here is the conceptualisation of the self as a body of water, one that loses its tranquillity due to illness. Such a perception of the self as a body of water can be traced to the literature and poetry of Iran after Islam. The Islamic symbology of water and the thoughts following from the framework defined by this symbology, has been further developed in the Iranian literature, and especially in the Mystic and Sufi poetry. In these works of literature water is seen as symbolising both the spirit of the human beings, as well as a purifying and cleansing entity. The association of water with the self follows from the symbol of water as the origin of all things, as well as the qualities of change and rebirth—of the soul more than the body—as seen in the ancient mythologies and the Islamic teachings. These symbols, in turn, have found their way into the everyday language of people and are often used in metaphorical forms to convey various messages.

One example of such portrayal of the self can be seen in Rumi's poetry. In his poetry, Rumi sees the human soul and mentality as a body of water, one that needs to be kept calm and tranquil, to keep it from physical and mental impurities (Obeydinia and Valinezhad 2009, p. 38). In other words, in this portrayal, one's health, as a body of water, is measurable by the calmness it enjoys, whereas the storminess and the waves of water can be seen as representative of a loss of balance and thus a symptom of ill health. This is to some extent in association with the way in which traditional Iranian medicine conceptualises ill health, namely as a loss of balance in the physical and mental forces. Depression, in this picture, is presented as disrupting the calmness of the self, turning the waters stormy and causing the imbalance in the mental life, and thus the perception of the self.

Metaphors of water, given the cultural ways of thinking that give rise to them, can be thought of as culture specific metaphors that cannot be seen as drawing on a basic universal conceptual metaphor. The cultural rootedness of these metaphors makes it difficult to see how, if at all, this way of thinking and talking about depression can be understood in terms of universal cognitive systems. It rather finds its meaning largely against the backdrop of cultural ways of thought and interpretations of the self and the world.

Culture-specific metaphors, in addition to drawing on cultural understandings and symbology, often draw on individual experiences and interpretations of these symbols, making it difficult to have a clear-cut way of interpreting the metaphors, in a way that is generalizable to the broader cultural context. The complexity of the use, and the messages conveyed by these metaphors, however, does not mean that they are unhelpful. On the contrary, they provide an insight into some of the ways in which people in Iran conceptualise themselves, depression, and their relation to depression, which in turn could be informative not only of their experiences of depression, but also their behaviours in response to it. For example, seeing patients articulating their experiences in terms of a metaphor, which is traceable to the traditional ways of conceptualising illness and health, could be informative about their help-seeking behaviours. This could be seen in Iranian patients' reluctance in seeking mainstream medication in treating their depression, and instead seeking traditional alternative remedies to alleviate their symptoms. Viewed in this way, the metaphorical language used in articulating experiences of depression, can point to significant differences in patients' responses to depression across cultures, as arising from cultural ways of thinking about and interpreting depression.

If we adopt a cognitive-linguistic framework for understanding metaphors, we also would have to accept that metaphors, their formation as well as their use, are rooted in conceptual frameworks for understanding and interpreting different phenomenon. As such, a study of metaphorical articulations of experiences of depression can offer a way of understanding depression that takes into account the different cultural ways of conceptualising and interpreting depression. In cases where the metaphors are widespread enough to be considered universal, one could argue that the cognitive framework of understanding the illness is shared across cultures. This assumption would also hold for metaphors which, despite their slight variation in form, are rooted in an identifiable underlying universal conceptual system. Nonetheless, for those metaphors that are deeply rooted in cultural ways of thought and interpretation, and thus irreducible to universal conceptual metaphors, the underlying cognitive framework would be unique to the culture in which these metaphors are formed and used. Furthermore, given the emphasis placed on experiences in the formation of conceptual metaphors in the cognitive-linguistic framework, it follows that in cases of (largely) universal metaphors, the underlying experiences are largely similar. On the other hand, metaphors that are unique to the cultural setting in which they are uttered, point to frameworks for understanding and interpreting experiences that are unique to that culture. In such cases, studying the use of metaphors offers a way of understanding cultural conceptions that in one way or another, can influence the individuals' experiences of depression, and their way of encountering it in light of cultural understandings.

4

Death-Consciousness and Absurdity

In this chapter I turn to some of the most common symptoms of depression among Iranian patients. As the shown in the introductory chapter, feelings of meaninglessness and absurdity (32.6%) and hopelessness (39.5%) are the most complained about symptoms of depression among the sample, while sadness, one of the most frequent symptoms in the UK is only complained about by 16% of Iranians. Although hopelessness is a key feature of experience of depression across the two cultures, I argue that in Iran such feelings are closely related to complaints of absurdity. The presence of these feelings of absurdity, as a point of divergence between experiences of depression in Iran and the UK, are in turn rooted in cultural and religious frames of thought dominant in Iranian culture. The key claim in this chapter is that a dominant culture of death-consciousness significantly affects experiences of depression and the way people interpret these experiences.

Inevitably, the experience of any sort of serious illness, as the closest one could get to a bridge between life and death, would be affected by one's attitudes towards death. Furthermore, depression brings about existential feelings that can serve to amplify thoughts of death, which in turn influence the way one experiences depression and responds to it. Given these observations, I will argue that certain symptoms and

M. Mirdamadi, *A Phenomenological Study of Depression in Iran*,
https://doi.org/10.1007/978-3-031-30407-1_4

manifestations of depression among Iranian patients can be analysed and accounted for through the examination of the death-conscious culture of Iran. These include the existence of a sense of absurdity with respect to oneself and one's life, as well as the different attitudes and responses towards suicide and suicidal thoughts. An analysis of this nature, in addition to accounting for the phenomenological significance of these experiences, also serves to explain the way in which these experiences vary due to cultural differences. In the first part of this chapter, I will outline what I mean by the culture of death-consciousness in Iran, as a pervasive way of understanding and relating to the world, before turning in the second part to the discussion of how this culture contributes to the variations in experiences of depression, as seen in Iran and the UK.

Iran as a Death-Conscious Culture

Schopenhauer identifies the 'denial of the will to live' with an ascetic attitude of renunciation and resignation, one that is reached by most people in proximity to death, in actuality but also in awareness and knowledge. He observes that this denial and the practices arising from it, are "further developed, more variously expressed, and more vividly presented, in the Sanskrit language than could be the case in the Christian church and the Western world" (Schopenhauer 1969, p. 387). He therefore points to a cultural difference between the East and the West, one characterised in terms of the extent of preoccupation with death; the death-conscious nature of the Eastern cultures (San'ati 2004).[1] Schopenhauer highlights these differences and praises the philosophy of life as practiced in the East, through mysticism and asceticism as the kind of practice that stays true to the nature of our being—with death as one of the pillars of this existence. Such a culture, manifestations of which

[1] Mohammad San'ati, a psychoanalyst and literary critic in Iran, claims that a broad range of behaviours seen among Iranians can be attributed to, and explained by, the observation of the culture as a death-conscious one (alternatively termed 'death culture') (San'ati 2004). This account is mostly brought out in terms of works of literature, and is aimed at explaining the everyday and routine behaviours of Iranians. Whilst borrowing the notion, I aim to give a more general understanding of the culture, and use it to account, specifically, for experiences of depression in Iran.

would be visible in various domains of life, religious and social practices alike, is phenomenologically significant, as it offers a way for articulating, understanding, and interpreting one's experiences. Indeed, preoccupations with death exist in every culture, as a universal human and existential concern. However, as I describe here, the nature of the relationship Iranians have with death, and its pervasiveness in the culture and cultural conceptualisations, distinguishes the death-conscious culture of the country from the broader concern with death which is seen universally across cultures.

The Iranian preoccupation with death, both as a physical end to the worldly life, as well as a gateway to heaven and hell, can be seen and traced in various cultural domains, including religious practices, works of literature and poetry, and social domains. The collective experiences of war and the devastating effects it has had on a large part of the population has also shaped, in large part, the existence of the culture of death-consciousness as presently seen in Iran. Although this collective experience itself has shaped a large part of the Iranian consciousness today, its continuing power in framing cultural ways of thought and interpretation is in part due to the pre-existing cultural and religious landscape in Iran. Furthermore, the Islamic Revolution of 1979 and the establishment that resulted from it are inseparable parts of this death-conscious culture. Being ideological in nature, it has had the power of directing this culture in a way that is pervasive throughout all aspects of one's being. This is seen clearly in the discourse of war, as well as the way religious elements of death-consciousness are taught in schools and talked about in mass media on a daily basis. Although the focus here is on historical and cultural roots of death-consciousness in Iran, the undeniable role of the governing regime ought to be borne in mind, as a powerful force in shaping the dominant culture and values in Iran today. It is, of course, important to note the variety in the approaches to understanding and encountering death in the Iranian culture. My argument, rather than implying that this form of death-consciousness is the only way of thinking about death in the Iranian culture, should be taken as highlighting that it is a dominant way of doing so. This dominance is due in part to the ideological nature of government which tends to highlight a particular narrative, and in part due to the recent history of Iran, which has further strengthened this narrative. As such, whilst this culture, due to its dominance and presence in the daily lives of Iranians, has a large influence on the common ways of thinking about death, it is by no means the sole narrative.[2]

Iran-Iraq War

As mentioned in Chap. 2, Iran went through one of the longest wars in the twentieth century with Iraq in the 1980s. The war started in September 1980, only a year after the Islamic Revolution which resulted in regime change in Iran, and went on for eight years until it ended in July 1988 following the United Nations Resolution for a ceasefire. The devastation of the war reached far beyond the border with Iraq and affected every single area of the country, following 'war of the cities', a bombing campaign by the Iraqi forces which targeted civilian areas to "help to break the enemy's will" (McNaugher 1990, p. 8). Such bombing campaigns were in addition to the use of chemical weapons on the Iranian population which killed many and caused lifelong injuries to many more. Official statistics by the Iranian Military, which were not published until 2015, estimate that a total of five million Iranians were directly involved in the war—including military, voluntary, and logistical forces. By the end of the war, 190 thousand were killed, 16 thousand of these during the bombing of residential areas, and the rest on the frontlines. Among the dead were 33 thousand school students and over 3.5 thousand university students. The number of those who suffered lifelong injuries, chemical or otherwise, stood at 672 thousand, while there were 42 thousand who were taken hostage and returned to Iran following the end of the war (TarikhIrani 2014). About 5 million of the population from the worst hit areas, were displaced and sought sanctuary in the central parts of the country.

[2] For instance, much of the mystic poetry and literature is seen as hopeful in the way it celebrates life. Yet this aspect can be overshadowed by the life-denying elements of these works due to, for example, the state-imposed censorship, preventing these elements to be brought out in the open as much as other aspects.

With the population boom in the country during the years of war, a large part of the current population of Iran was either born or spent a significant part of their childhood during the war. The traumatic experiences of war, and the memories which remain in the collective consciousness of this generation, such as the sounds of the sirens warning of airstrikes and urging citizens to take shelter underground, remains part of the generational sense of identity of the young population of Iran (e.g. Behrouzan 2016). As such, the experiences of war, rather than limited to those who fought at the frontlines, affected everyone living through it.

Additionally, as noted earlier, government policies in place since the war act not only to keep the memories of war alive, but also to sanctify the horrors of the war. Tales of those killed and injured continue to be part of the compulsory school curricula, while their giant murals remain visible on the face of different cities in Iran. Streets and alleys in every town across the country are named after those who lost their lives in the war. And for those who disappeared in the warfronts or were never identified, streets are named as '*shahid-e gomnām*' or 'unnamed martyr'. The dominant discourse continues to sanctify the horrors of war: it is not a 'war', but 'The Holy Defence', and those killed are not 'casualties' but 'martyrs'. Various national ceremonies aim at keeping the stories and memories of the lives lost alive. In addition to such efforts, the traumatic experiences of the war continue to haunt, not only those families whose children's remains were never found and for whom loss remains a timeless pain, but the whole nation. People continue to lose their lives in minefields which are yet to be fully cleared (BBC Persian 2017). In 2015, the bodies of 175 divers who had been taken captive in 1986 were found, after they were buried alive over thirty years earlier, and as recently as September 2017, the remains of a 13-year-old boy, killed in the war was returned to Iran to be buried after 34 years.

The memories of war and its traumatic experiences, centred around death and lost lives, far from representing an event in the distant past, are part of the daily routines and preoccupations of Iranians, and continue to shape people's lives, thoughts and feelings. Not only do the memories continue to haunt those who experienced the war, but even for those born after the end of the war, the wounds and the aftereffects of it remain a tangible force. One of these effects, I argue, is the relationship Iranians have with death, as something always near and always looming. Arguably, with the immense shared sense of loss, and with daily reminders of death, this relationship with death goes a step further than the existential feeling every human being, regardless of their culture and society, is preoccupied with in their lives. This constant awareness and consciousness of death, as seen in Iranian society today, however, despite being amplified by the effects of war and the devastation it has inevitably brought, and which has lasted for years after its end, is also traceable to other elements of Iranian culture with a much longer history. It is the combination of historical context and current sense of life and experiences that gives rise to the culture of death-consciousness in Iran.

Shi'ite Teachings

It is widely thought that in religious societies, fear and anxiety towards death is considerably lower than non-religious societies (e.g. Soenke et al. 2013; Koenig 2009), due to the comfort gained through faith in the afterlife and the existence of a realm beyond the physical one inhabited during one's life. However, a tension can be observed in some of the religious teachings and conceptualisations of death. While these often involve the reassurance that death is not an end but simply a gateway to another, more permanent realm closer to God, believers are simultaneously invited to be aware and fearful of death in every instance of their lives. This dichotomous portrayal of the notion of death and how one ought to relate to it, could lead to a confusion that could further enflame the anxieties people feel towards death. The teachings of Shi'ism, for example, serve to show this tension.

One of the most important texts in the teachings of Shi'ism is Nahj ul-Balagha, the collection of letters and sermons attributed to Ali, the first Imam for Shi'a Muslims, and the cousin of Prophet Mohammad. As noted in Chap. 2, for Iranians Ali embodies the ideal character, with all virtues attributed to him. Seen by Iranians as a role model, then, it is not surprising that Nahj ul-Balagha, which encompasses his teachings and thoughts, both on religious matters but more generally about how one ought to think about oneself and one's life and the best way for living this life, has remained one of the most important texts in Shi'ism and one that Iranians adhere to. The notion of death and the individual's relation to it is one of the topics covered extensively in these teachings, so much so that this particular text is considered to put forward one of the most important narratives of death in Shi'ite thought (Nejati Hosseini 2013). The teachings regarding death in this text cover a wide range of issues including the fear of death, the inescapability of death, the constant remembering and the impossibility of forgetting death and death as the end of one's (physical) life.

One of the most important points of emphasis in this text, is the necessity of 'death-consciousness' (*marg-āgāhi*). It is argued that this way of being offers a way for the believer to "know themselves, and in turn, find a way of understanding the meaning of life" (Taheri Sarteshnizi and Moosavi 2012, p. 177—my translation). On this point, the life of a person who has forgotten death, and in turn has forgotten the afterlife, is likened to the state of the one walking in complete darkness, lost and led astray by the darkness (Letter No. 31). Such a person should be reminded that "with death, the darkness is removed and the truths [of the world] are illuminated" (Taheri Sarteshnizi and Moosavi 2012, p. 180—my translation). Thus, it is claimed that remembering death at every living moment, would in fact give one a better understanding of the world and how one ought to live in it. This kind of encouragement is further justified through ethical obligations and the encouragement to be good. The belief in a heaven and hell, as the eternal place for reward or punishment based on the actions one commits in this world, act both as an encouragement to be good, and a deterrent for doing bad. Since in the Islamic teachings, our life is merely a preparation for the afterlife, the belief in the immanency of death serves as a reminder for the believers that they need to do good, as there might not be time to make up for any bad or unethical deeds they commit. As such, there are short bold reminders of the immanency of death in this text: "anticipate your death by good actions … and prepare yourselves for death, since it is hovering over you" (Sermon No.64).

In illuminating the true meaning of life, consciousness of death also serves as a reminder of the illusory value we tend to attach to material things that bring us joy, or otherwise present themselves as valuable. This again can be understood through the portrayal of this world and our lives in it. As the Islamic teachings hold, this world is merely a passageway to the afterlife, and is a means of preparation for the good life one could lead in the more permanent afterlife. Meanwhile, this world is portrayed as deceptive, with various material things or events that could distract one from the main aim, that is, preparation for the afterlife. As such, remembering death, is in a sense a reminder of the life awaiting the believer and can serve as a preventive force against the distractions of the material world: "surely the remembrance of death has kept me away from fun and play while obliviousness about the next world has prevented him from speaking truth" (Sermon No. 84).

In this latter justification of death consciousness, another element closely linked with it is manifest, namely the denial of earthly pleasures and joyous acts and things, since these are construed as distractions from the real values and the real meaning of life. This element of denial of life, in the face of awareness of death is in itself noteworthy in the process of viewing life as inherently meaningless and absurd, which is heightened in depression due to the existential change it brings about. If there is already a strong disposition dominant in the religious culture against attachment to joys and pleasures of life, then in the face of depression, this disposition could come to the foreground, bringing the motivation and process for feeling joyous again in life and freeing oneself from depression into question. The religious teachings of Shi'ism (and especially in Islamic mysticism which dominate some of the most important literary works of Iran), are filled with such claims regarding the value we tend to mistakenly attach to the material things. This lengthy, but important part of a Sermon in Nahj ul-Balagha can serve as an example of this thinking:

> Certainly this world is a dirty watering place and a muddy source of drinking. Its appearance is attractive and its inside is destructive. It is a deception, a vanishing reflection and a bent pillar. When its despiser begins to like it and he who is not acquainted with it feels satisfied with it, then it raises and puts down its feet (in joy), entraps him in its trap, makes him the target of its arrows and puts round his neck the rope of death taking him to the narrow grave and fearful abode in order to show him his place of stay and the recompense of his acts. This goes on from generation to generation. Neither death stops from cutting them asunder nor do the survivors keep aloof from committing of sins. (Sermon No. 83)

There are various other examples from the Islamic, and in particular Shi'ite teachings that encourage consciousness of death and embracing death rather than life. However, the emphasis placed on the notion of death in Iranian culture is not limited to the religious texts and teaching, but is also found in old and recent works of Iranian literature.

Iranian Literature

The preoccupation with death in the Iranian literature can be traced back to the twelfth century to poets from the mystic tradition such as Rumi, Attar and Omar Khayyam. Islamic mysticism, and in particular Iranian Sufism, emphasises the importance of the spiritual message of Islam and "attempt to live the modalities of this message in a personal way through the interiorization of the content of the Quranic Revelation" (Corbin 2014, p. 187). As such, in the poetry inspired by this tradition, the personal experience and relation with God and God's religion is emphasised. Reflecting this deep personal relationship, the concern with death as the ultimate bridge that would bring the Sufi and God together, as well as the question of life and how one ought to think about the dichotomy of life and death, are explored extensively in the Sufi literature and poetry. Given the spiritual nature of these practices and traditions, they reflect the denial of earthly pleasures and attachment to them, as seen in the Shi'ite teachings, while at the same time highlighting the inevitability of death and the important role it plays (or should play) in the way one conducts oneself.

In his *Masnavi*, which is one of the most important and influential works in Sufism, Rumi extensively talks about the awareness of death and how this awareness ought to play a part in what we consider to be the right way of life. One example of this is the story of The Arab and His Wife. In the story, the Wife speaks out complaining about the sufferings of their family, due to being poor and not having enough to enjoy their lives: "How very poor we are! What hardships have we borne! The whole world lives in pleasures; we're the butt of scorn!" (Rumi 1881/1273, p. 220). The response from the Arab, is one emphasising that such anxieties and sufferings are portions of death, reminding them that the pleasures of life are only temporary and that in order to live a good life and afterlife, these sufferings are necessary:

> All those anxieties that fall on us like darts,
> Are but the vapours, tempests, of our human hearts.
> Those cares are like a sickle, made to cut us down.
> This is a fact, though we are slow the truth to own.
> …
> Our troubles are the heralds of our death to come.
> Turn not thy face away from herald, as do some.
> Whoever leads a joyous life finds death severe.
> And he who's slave to body, mars his soul's career.
> When sheep come home from pasture in the meadows green,
> The fattest ones are slaughtered, soon as they are seen. (Ibid., p. 222)

What is striking about the portrayal of death and one's relation to it in this passage, is the association of all earthly sufferings with death and awareness of it; just as death is inevitable, so is suffering in this world. And, furthermore, if one is wise, one ought to embrace this suffering, since denying it would amount to denial of death as a necessary element of life, and thus ultimately living a lie. In contrast, the more one embraces the suffering in this world, whatever form it takes—recall that being good is always associated with having to suffer, and good people necessarily endure immense suffering—an easier and 'sweeter' death and afterlife will be rewarded.

Attar's portrayal of death is also along the same lines, albeit put more boldly and clearly. In *The Conference of the Birds* (~1177), Attar states that we are all born just to die and despite our attachment to the joys of life, these are merely trivialities in the face of death, and this is clear to anyone who is aware of death. And furthermore, he states that the only cure from death is death itself, as seen in the following extract from *A viceroy at the point of death*:

> The man replied, 'except that every day
> I lived was wasted on what's trivial,
> And now I shall be dust -- and that is all.'

> To seek death is death's only cure -- the leaf
> Grows hectic and must fall; our life is brief.
> Know we are born to die; the soul moves on;
> The heart is pledged and hastens to be gone.
> ...
> Look hard at death -- in our long pilgrimage
> The grave itself is but the first grim stage;
> How your sweet life would change if you could guess
> The taste of death's unequalled bitterness. (Attar 1984/1177)

These examples from the classical period of Persian poetry (twelfth to thirteenth century), show the way these giants of poetry viewed and responded to the notion of death, as a source of anxiety and fear, but also a notion that ought to be recognized and embraced in order to lead a good life. Both of these elements of the notion of death can be traced to the religious teachings and the dominant frame of thought and interpretation of the time. Preoccupation with death continues to be the subject of many works of literature through to the modern times, although with a refined attitude towards it.

In the contemporary setting, and with the focus shifting from religious thought into a more socially concerned attitude, the concern with death is framed with reference to dissatisfaction and even hatred of life itself. One of the poets in this time, whose thoughts on the interplay of life and death is clearly articulated in his work, is Mehdi Akhavan-Sales. For Akhavan, poetry was a way of fighting mortality (San'ati 2013, p. 152), and in many of his poems his frustration is clear to the extent that he proclaims, many times, his hatred of life. He points to the pointless repetition of life, sees life as "this futile, this fearful darkness" (Life, 1966—my translation), and calls the pointless days following on from one another as "remaining futile and empty and filthy" (Mordāb, 1978—my translation), and even more distinctly, he says of life: "I have seen for a lifetime its ups and downs, [I] spit on its face, damn its meaning" (Again, One Must Live, 1979—my translation). Despite this clear frustration with life, Akhavan also says that he loves life, pointing to an internal polarity, and this is where, for him, death comes into play:

I see life as friend,
death as enemy
Oh! But with whom can I say this,
I have a friend
From whom I want to take shelter and turn to the enemy (As a Thirsty Urn, 1959—my translation)

The striking turn seen here, compared to the earlier poetry, with regards to death, is one where death-consciousness is not encouraged as a way of being good or leading a good life, but rather, death is seen as desirable in the face of the difficulty, absurdity, and even the injustices of life. Death is seen as the ultimate shelter from life itself. This way of thinking about death was seen earlier in the works of Sadegh Hedayat, from whom Akhavan also took immense inspiration (San'ati 2013).

What is shared between Hedayat and Akhavan, and many other modern writers and poets, is the critical attitude they take towards the issues in socio-political and cultural domains, and the way their writing is in sync with their personal experiences of these issues. It is through such experiences and their close study and awareness of the socio-political, as well as the cultural developments of their time in Iran, that their work is formed and the struggles are articulated. In this change of tone and points of concern, Hedayat was one of the first intellectuals in Iran who wrote about and criticised the dominant cultural attitudes and norms, and a lack of critical reflection on these in the Iranian society. Some of the cultural attitudes Hedayat was concerned with were those concerned with death; he was critical of these attitudes which in his mind deny the reality of death as the end of one's being, while at the same time, pronouncing his dissatisfaction with life and his desire to escape from it. In Hedayat's writings, as in Akhavan's, one sees this tension between hating life and being fearful of death, suffering in life and awaiting death, whilst at the same time being critical of the way death and death consciousness have been encouraged in the culture. There is love for life but longing for death, both playing a part in their writings. This is seen in the famous opening of *The Blind Owl* where Hedayat writes: "There are certain sores in life that, like a canker, gnaw at the soul in solitude and diminish it" (Hedayat 1974/1934). It is this kind of sores, these sufferings in life which, for Hedayat, act as a drive towards voluntary death, despite a deep fear of death. Sufferings which make life itself seem unworthy of living and death as the ultimate saviour.

Hedayat was one of the first Iranian writers and intellectuals who not only was familiar with Western nihilism, but who also used this knowledge in his writings. The influence of French thinkers and writers, as well as other European thinkers such as Freud, and writers such as Kafka, is evident in his writings. It is in Hedayat's works that the first instance of talking of absurdity of life and living is seen in the domain of Iranian literature. *The Blind Owl*, as his most celebrated piece of writing—also considered the most important work of Iranian literature in the twentieth century—embodies Hedayat's unique attitude to life and death. This is also because the Blind Owl, the narrator of the story, is supposed to represent Hedayat himself with all his points of concern and attitudes. 'The sores that gnaw at the soul', for Hedayat (or for the Blind Owl) represent an unresolvable dichotomy; the social and cultural reasons and ways of life that bind one "because he cannot go further than the line drawn for him" (Hedayat 1948, p. 13—my translation), but also "a closed condemnation that follows [him], that his encounter is only with absurdity (*pooch*) and the absurdity is the shallow and mortal life, thus the acceptance of the final nothingness" (San'ati 2015, p. 7—my translation). This tension, being condemned to be face to face with the inevitable nothingness of life whilst being unable to escape from it, creates an existential anxiety that is manifest in Hedayat's writings, and results in a turn to death. As Sanati puts it, "if this existential anxiety dazzled Kafka in an animal depersonalisation, caused Sartre nausea and drifted Camus into alienation and estrangement, for a mentality like Hedayat's, it brought suffocation and death" (Ibid.—my translation).

It is in the face of this anxiety, that in the course of *The Blind Owl*, the reader sees that the desire to live slowly disappears in the protagonist "and what consoles him is the hope of nothingness after death" (San'ati 2015, p. 54—my translation), whilst alongside this hope for nothingness, the paralysing fear of death grows and adds to the anxiety of his every living moment. *The Blind Owl* is written on the basis of the dichotomy and the contrast between life and death, and the anxiety arising from this dichotomy is further strengthened by the opposition of Good and Evil, the contrasting forces dominant in the Iranian culture and society that limit the power of the Blind Owl to act and the constant remembering of which adds to his anxiety. The interplay of these various forces is striking in the novel, and the symbolism revealing the connection between these forces needs careful attention to be fleshed out. One such example is the character of Blind Owl's wife (and cousin), who symbolises a "transcendental unloving", and symbolises for the Blind Owl the world and life within it: "a death-inducing world in which one is always standing on the edge of the cliff of nothingness, and where relationships are unstable, and death is the manifestation of this unloving" (San'ati 2015, p. 213– my translation).

The Blind Owl remains the subject of various studies, psychological and sociological, as well as literary ones. But it also remains the first serious work in Iranian literature that talks boldly not only of death, but also fear of death, the absurdity of life in the face of this inevitable end, whilst criticising the way this notion is construed culturally and socially, and is thus largely influential. This influence is seen in the works of writers and poets that came after Hedayat, as has been seen in the works of Akhavan-Sales. What further adds to the influence of this work, is Hedayat's own carefully thought-out suicide which, among speculations and debates, has further brought his works and thoughts into the public domain. Many have argued that Hedayat was visibly depressed, and his suicide serves as evidence to this point. This argument, regardless of whether it is true (and many would argue that it is not), has helped the association of Hedayat's thoughts and writings with depression; some would even go as far as framing their experiences in terms of Hedayat's thoughts. Because of this perceived advocacy for absurdist thinking and suicide, for years, and especially after the Islamic Revolution in Iran, Hedayat and his works, in particular *The Blind Owl*, have been pushed to the side, dismissed as unworthy, censored and at times banned from being republished. There are some "who try so hard to portray him as a monster and a dangerous person who had nothing to do but to think about absurdity, bitterness, misfortune, and suicide. And thus adamantly try to erase him from the history of Iranian literature and do not mention his name in the media and advise young people not to read him, even if it is only to save their lives" (Masoodiniya 2017—my translation). Despite such efforts, not only does Hedayat remain one of the most well-known authors in Iran, but also the thoughts and frustrations he portrays in his work, remain an integral part of Iranian culture and society and so his works act as a reference point for many who feel similar frustrations.

Death-Conscious Culture and Depression

The existence of a death-conscious culture in Iran, and its place in cultural conceptualisations and the dominant discourse in society, have a demonstrable influence on manifestations of depression among Iranian patients. In what follows, I examine this effect on attitudes towards suicide and suicidal thoughts and the kind of responses people have to these in light of the death-conscious culture, before turning to depressive symptoms, such as feelings of hopelessness and the way patients' articulations and experiences of these symptoms are informed by this pre-existing culture. Through this analysis it can be seen that certain variations in experiences of depression between Iran and the UK can be accounted for through the difference in individuals' relation with death.

Death-Consciousness and Suicide

In Iran, as elsewhere, depressed patients are preoccupied with thoughts of death and suicide:

#4(F) – The world seems fake (*alaki*) and like a game and I wish my life would end sooner.

#6(F) – I suddenly get free (*rahā*) of all mental and emotional bounds (*ta'alogh*) and I only want not to be. Although I always prefer not being, to being, but in episodes of depression I think about it more and get closer to it.

#7(F) – [I] wish I would die. How long do I have to suffer here. To what end (*ākharesh ke chi*)? All levels of life are pointless and it ends in the end there is death!

#10(F) – [In depression] the feeling of death becomes stronger in me.
#16(F) – I think depression is a lack of desire to continue life.
#20(F) – I feel I have had enough of life and want to end my life and die.
FB#1 – Most of the time I think about death [and] I feel a big sense of emptiness inside me.

Suicide is considered to be a cardinal sin in Islam, and in various religious texts it is seen as grounds for a long or even an eternal punishment. For example, in the Quran, it is said "…Nor kill (or destroy) yourselves: for God hath been to you most Merciful! If any do that in rancour or injustice, soon shall we cast them into the fire" (The Quran, 4.29–30).[3] In a sermon attributed to Imam Sadiq, the sixth Imam of Shi'ite Muslims, it is also emphasised that whoever knowingly kills himself, will forever be in the fires of hell (Al-Koleini 1990). This standing of suicide in religious teachings has multiple influences. In Iran, with an ideological religious state in place, although suicide is not an illegal act, there is a noticeable lack of research, quantitative and qualitative, on suicide. To protect its image as an Islamic country no reliable statistics on rates of suicide are collected, since acknowledgement of the phenomenon would imply the existence of people disregarding religious rules prohibiting suicide.

In the absence of such statistics, it is difficult to say in general terms what attitude Iranians take towards suicide. However, certain factors, such as the culture of death-consciousness which sometimes amounts to denial of life, as well as the struggles of patients diagnosed with depression with social stigmas and lack of societal empathy (examined in Chaps. 6 and 7), make it plausible that suicide rates in Iran would be high. Although such a claim would be difficult to justify using statistical evidence, scattered first-person and eye-witness accounts suggest that at least the rates of suicide attempts, regardless of whether they are successful or not, is high. In a newspaper article in October 2016, for example, the reporter writes about a night in an emergency room for poisoning at a

[3] The point regarding suicide appears alongside stealing and consuming another's wealth 'unjustly'. The 'rancour or injustice' referred to here, can be in reference to the earlier line. Equally it could refer to suicide: since God as the creator of all individuals knows best when to start and end a life, taking the matters in one's own hands is seen as an aggressive act of injustice to the pre-determined order of the world.

hospital in central Tehran. In the twelve hours between 8pm and 8am, 33 people were brought into the emergency room, 26 of whom had attempted suicide by taking pills and/or poison (Samgis 2016). All of those admitted to the hospital for attempted suicide were aged 16–40 and most of them had a history of psychiatric illness. The interviews with the staff at the emergency room suggests that such rate of suicide attempts was common in that hospital.

This report suggests that suicide attempts in Iran may be more common among younger people. In 2020 and with the emotional and economic difficulties brought about by the pandemic, numerous reports of suicide among younger Iranians emerged. Official accounts of reasons of these suicides range from mental disorders to family issues and it is difficult to know what motivates such acts (Mirdamadi 2021). If those who attempt suicide in Iran do tend to be younger, this would be in line with global trends—based on the World Health Organization's findings, suicide is the second leading cause of death among 15–29 year olds globally (World Health Organization 2018). But in addition, any difference in Iran might be a manifestation of a division between religiosity in different generational groups, which leads to different attitudes and interpretations of the death-conscious culture of Iran.

Notably, the older generation tend to have stronger religious beliefs which adhere to a more literal reading of religious teachings, as compared to the younger generation. Those adhering to the more literal reading of religious teachings are more likely to avoid committing suicide. Instead, as a psychiatrist in Iran has told me, patients suffering from depression in Iran, due to their religious beliefs which prohibit taking one's own life, often resort to what is termed 'passive suicide'. This consists in praying for God to end and take one's life, rather than acting themselves and taking the matter in their own hands. In other words, although almost all depressed patients are occupied with suicidal thoughts, given their fear of God, and following the Islamic teachings, which see suicide as one of the cardinal sins, the majority would rather not act upon these thoughts themselves (Moghimi 2017, personal correspondence). Asking God to take their lives would mean they have fulfilled their wish to die to an extent by articulating their thoughts and desires to an all-powerful Being, whilst at the same time circumventing committing a punishable sin and going against their faith and beliefs.

On the other hand, those for whom the faith and belief in various religious teachings are not as strong, death-consciousness would more easily translate to suicidal thoughts that potentially initiate action. The prevalence of a more individualistic approach to religion, which leaves space for personal interpretations of the religious values and teachings has been increasing and is now common among the younger generation in Iran (e.g. Alamzadeh and Rastegari 2015; Shojaeizand et al. 2006). Whilst those who take the literal readings of religion to heart would be more prepared to accept as given the teachings of Islam by a religious expert/cleric, those with a more interpretive and individualistic attitude to religion are more sceptical and tend to project their own values and personal feelings and experiences on the religious values and teachings. For example, one might accept prima facie that suicide is sinful, yet argue that each individual is the one responsible for how her life develops and ends. In the face of immense suffering, therefore, it would not be uncommon to hear reasoning along the lines that 'even God would not want to see me suffer in this way'. Or, one might choose to prioritise other teachings over those that condemn suicide, and argue that, for example, the fact that God is all-forgiving takes precedence over suicide being a cardinal sin.

One important observation that needs to be acknowledged here is the role of religious beliefs in individuals' wellbeing. It is generally accepted that religious beliefs have a positive role to play in wellbeing; one's happiness and satisfaction of life, as well as hopefulness and optimism (Van Ness and Larson 2002). However, the relationship between religiosity and fear and anxieties in the face of death, is less straightforward (e.g. Thorson and Powell 1988, 1990). As can be seen from various studies done in Iran, "religion acts as a protection and improvement in the state of acceptance and readiness towards one's own or another's death" (Nejati Hosseini 2013, p. 42—my translation). Simultaneously, religion itself can be a factor contributing to fear of death. In a 2014 study, which examines the reasons and elements contributing to fear of death, the largest factor was found to be "pain and punishment in the afterlife", with "failure to do religious duties" as a reason highly correlated with belief in religious teachings (Aflakseir 2014, pp. 25–26). In other words, whilst everyone taking part in the study identified the afterlife as a main cause of their fear of death, those who held religious beliefs, saw failure to do what is required by their beliefs, arguably another manifestation of their fear of punishment in the afterlife, as the main reason for their sensed fear of death. As such, the argument presented here, in so far as it is concerned with anxieties arising from awareness of death as encouraged by religious teachings, rather than consolations received about these anxieties from religion, remains valid.

Death-Consciousness and Depressive Symptoms

Certain symptoms and manifestations of depression seen in Iran, including feelings of hopelessness and absurdity, can be closely linked with the death-conscious culture. While some degree of hopelessness seems to be a universal part of the experience of depression, the questionnaire results suggest a higher emphasis placed on loss of hope among Iranian patients. In fact, hopelessness is central to the Iranian experience of depression to the extent that often patients define depression itself in terms of hopelessness.

#3(F) – I think depression has a strong correlation with hope, losing hope/becoming hopeless for whatever reason in my opinion is depression.

#14(F) – In my opinion depression is the feeling of hopelessness and despair, which causes one to become incapable of doing the normal daily tasks.

Ratcliffe argues that the sense of hopelessness in depression is rooted in the existential change involved in depression, since the *existential* loss of hope in depression is fundamentally different, and phenomenologically stronger than the *intentional* hopelessness one might feel in everyday situations (Ratcliffe 2015). As an intentional state, intentional hope is *about* something in the world; I hope *that* event x happens. Similarly, losing hope for event x can be construed as no longer having the intentional state of hope, for a certain event x. What defines existential loss of hope, Ratcliffe argues, is the transformation of one's space of possibilities into one of impossibility, where hoping for a state of affairs to come to be becomes essentially irrational, since the very possibility of the desirable state of affairs is under question.

While I agree with this characterisation of hopelessness in depression, I would argue that one needs to say more about how this process of transformation of space of possibilities into one of impossibility is brought about and how individuals respond to this transformation. In the case of Iranian patients, I would argue this process is intimately linked with the Iranian conceptualisations of life and depression, whilst the responses to this transformation are connected with thoughts and practices of death-consciousness.

#14(F) – I saw the world as uncertain (*mobham*), and full of hopelessness and despair (*ya'as*).
#25(M) – [When depressed] the world has no meaning for me and I'm not hopeful about life.
#28(F) – My depression has caused me to be dispirited about life and has caused me to continue life with hopelessness.
#15(F) – Depression means moodiness (*bi-hoselegi*), restlessness, hopelessness.

There are two elements at play here, understanding both of which is essential in understanding the feelings of hopelessness in depressed patients in Iran and the emphasis placed on this feeling as a central symptom of depression; namely, the Iranian conceptions of life itself, and the cultural conceptualisations of depression. As discussed in Chap. 2, the common conceptions of depression in Iran often attribute the cause of depression to an outside source, out of the control of the individual. As such, there is often an element of dissatisfaction with the world in which one dwells and a sense of one being a victim of these outside influences. In such a conception, one's efforts in taking control of one's life and protecting oneself against the outside influences are felt to have been in vain—and it is through the realisation of this effort in vain that depression comes about. Depression, from its conception to its manifestations as seen in Iran, seems to be the embodiment of the struggles of each individual against the world, and one which is, to a certain extent, the logical place these struggles lead to.[4] This latter point is closely connected with the Iranian conceptions of life as fundamentally a fight, a struggle to strike a balance between the forces of Good and Evil. In other words, the feelings of dissatisfaction and the sense of being a victim in the world can be thought of as the expression of the inherently unfair fight one is made to endure. In this sense, depression is thought of as the logical ending point, once one realises the nature of this unfair fight. Once one is fallen into depression, and due to the existential change one goes through in depression, which transforms one's perception of oneself and of one's world, the sense of helplessness becomes overwhelming, and it is in such a situation where any hope for change and a move forward is lost. The very hope, that is, which up until this point would have fuelled the ongoing fight forward. The existential hopelessness in depression, then, brings into question the very meaning of life as a fight to be fought, and is therefore the hopelessness of even envisioning a change, and conceiving of an improvement in one's life—no hope is left for even fantasising about a different world. This, I believe, is the impossibility Iranian depressed patients are faced with, one which, in altering the individual's perceptions, brings into question the meaning of life and the motivation to strive forwards.

This could further present an account of the way in which one's space of possibilities is transformed into impossibility as a result of the existential change one goes through in depression. Once understood, this process can also illuminate the heavy emphasis placed on feelings of hopelessness among Iranian patients, as the defining symptom of depression. It follows from the arguments above, that the rootedness of this feeling in the Iranian culture and conceptions gives this feeling the importance and centrality that is expressed by those suffering from depression.

[4] It could be argued that the hopelessness felt and talked about so often among Iranians, can be thought of as an idiom of distress, one which finds its expression in depression: depression is the means through which these pre-existing thoughts and feelings are expressed. I will look at this proposition in Chap. 8.

Importantly, however, (and the way in which the feelings of hopelessness in Iranian depressive patients is distinguished from those in the UK), is the role of the culture of death-consciousness already prevalent in Iran, and its influences on the feelings of hopelessness. Specifically of importance here are the accounts of life and death as presented in the literature of twentieth century Iran. As shown above, in such works of literature, the message conveyed is one in which the dissatisfaction with one's life, and a sense of having lost in the fight for a good life, forces one to come face to face with death as the ultimate end. Shown clearly in the poem by Akhavan, death becomes the only conceivable change, and thus the only goal one is able to hang onto. Death in such a scenario would be the only place one could take shelter from the hopelessness of life: death becomes the only remaining hope. This pre-existing culture which encourages the remembering of death both paves the way for this form of hopelessness, and offers a way of interpreting and understanding, and thus articulating one's feelings of frustration and dissatisfaction. This existential hopelessness, therefore, places more emphasis on death, as the only possibility amidst the impossibilities of life. This form of hopelessness, one that forces one to remember death in such a way, is further strongly connected with another feeling expressed by Iranian patients, namely absurdity.

#26(F) – I feel a sense of absurdity (*poochi*), nothing is interesting for me.
#21(F) – I feel a sense of absurdity and feel as if nothing is right and everything is a lie.
#9(F) – I think the world has no attractions even in the moment. Merely passing time and life without anything else.
#35(F) – I feel sadness and sorrow and [a sense of] absurdity.
#36(F) – I feel that the world is completely absurd and futile
#41(F) – Depression means feeling absurdity, and life becoming meaningless.

A linguistic point is worth making here regarding the meaning and connotation of the words used in this instance. The word used by Iranians, *poochi* (noun), which I have translated as absurdity, is derived from the adjective *pooch* which itself carries various meanings and heavy connotations. Among the dictionary meanings of *pooch* are empty, hollow, pointless, futile, nothingness, nonsensical, and lacking in meaning. Given these definitions, then, it can be seen that what Iranians mean in talking about feelings of absurdity or *poochi* in depression, is an expression of the way they see the world and themselves in it. Furthermore, given these meanings, the link between this expression and those of hopelessness become clear, since they are both rooted in the Iranian conceptualisations of life. The feelings of absurdity in this sense, emphasise the feelings of defeat and meaninglessness with regards to the fight which is life.

Now with the preceding account of hopelessness, where consciousness of death plays a central role, and where death itself is highlighted as the ultimate inescapable end, this sense of meaninglessness and emptiness of the world comes to the foreground: nothing can change the fact that death is inescapable. The depressed patient who is overwhelmed by the feelings of existential hopelessness is confronted with this fact, and as a result, any attempt to fight this inescapable end is seen as meaningless, since one can never win the ultimate fight with death. This latter point overshadows, and makes meaningless any effort for improvement, giving one's life and the world in which one dwells a quality of emptiness and absurdity. Various writers and thinkers have spoken of the inherent absurdity of life, but the sense of absurdity talked about by Iranians suffering from depression finds its meaning against the cultural conceptions of life as a meaningful fight. It is the sense of loss of meaning in depression, shaped by a sense of hopelessness against a death-conscious culture that is emphasised in complaints of absurdity among Iranians. One can see parallels here between these feelings of meaninglessness of the world, and the metaphors used by Iranians in talking about their experiences of depression, seen in Chap. 3. As argued before, the image of a colourless world signifies an idle and meaningless state in which no change can be envisioned and thus any attempt at improving one's state or hoping for a better future is seen as futile and absurd. Taken together, the metaphors of colour and the feelings of hopelessness and absurdity, make the argument for the existence of these feelings, as the defining features of depression in Iran, stronger.

Furthermore, these feelings of absurdity as felt in depression can in effect place into question one's previous understandings of oneself and one's life:

#3(F) – I am hopeless and at the same time feel absurdity (*poochi*) with regards to my life in the past, present and the future

As if in receipt of a higher understanding, the feelings of absurdity and hopelessness, in the face of consciousness of death, force one to think about the way one has led one's life up to this point and all previous conceptions of life and the world. Death is a sublime which makes one realise one's own mortality and insignificance and such feelings further force one to rethink how one has conducted oneself throughout one's life, and it all seems meaningless, empty, and absurd.

Additionally, following the earlier discussions from the religious teachings which encourage the remembering of death as a preventive force against the earthly joys of life, this feeling of absurdity and the meaninglessness of life in depression, can affect the behaviours patients have in response to depression. The tendency to deny life, brought to the foreground in light of the feelings of the absurdity of life, could in instances dampen the motivation to seek help. The unwillingness of the patients to find help and an effective treatment, presents a challenge for mental-health professionals. Looking at such issues in psychotherapy in particular, San'ati notes, in societies such as Iran, individuals "are prepared to use modern psychotherapies as modern cures, but they have been nurtured with a culture of death which is there, at least, in the back of their mind, challenging therapeutic attempts for change" (San'ati 2004). Such resistance, and the view of change as futile and meaningless, can further be explained through the conceptualisation of every suffering as 'a portion of death', and therefore as inevitable as death itself. If the suffering as a result of depression is conceptualised in this way, and if, as a result of the feelings brought about by depression, the thought of death and its conceptualisations in the culture is brought to the fore of one's attention, then one might see this suffering as necessary, to be embraced rather than treated and gotten rid of. In instances where these various elements are seen to be in play together, the unwillingness to seek help and treatment can be explained against the backdrop of the cultural conceptualisations of death and death-consciousness.

The exposition presented provides an example of where the dominant culture and the cultural ways of thought and interpretation influence the experiences of depression and shape the manifestations of depression. The death-conscious culture of Iran is manifested and conceptualised in different cultural elements and cemented through collective experiences and the dominant discourse of the state. The attitudes encouraged by this culture are heavily influential in the way Iranians conceptualise themselves and their lives, and their relation to the world in which they dwell and are therefore phenomenologically significant. Whilst I concede that many of these mechanisms and frameworks remain largely unconscious, an examination of the dominant forces of influence in the culture demonstrates the pervasiveness of such cultural modes of thought and interpretation. By bringing these mechanisms and frameworks to the foreground of consciousness, whilst acknowledging the fact that experiences find meaning against the backdrop of culture and dominant ways of thought, the role played by such mechanisms in shaping parts of experiences of depression within the culture are demonstrated.

5

Interpersonal Relationships I: Impersonal Interpersonal

An important and universal part of experiences of depression is its influence on interpersonal relationships. This influence, manifested in the breakdown of the interpersonal bond, can be seen in different domains of relations with others; namely one's relation with the indefinite, collective, 'impersonal' others, as well as one's relations with specific, determinate, 'personal' Others. I suggest that although the breakdown of the interpersonal bond can be thought of as a universal part of experiences of depression, the manifestations of the breakdown can be culturally specific, and in accordance with cultural norms and conceptualisations that govern our relations with others.

In Iran, as a collectivist society, often the boundaries between the social and the private, and the norms governing relationships in the two spheres, are blurred. In such a society, the experiences and goals of the individual are seen to be in the service of the collective, whilst the collective force of the society in setting the norms and dominant ways of being, remains powerful in the private spheres of life. As such, one of the complications when analysing a phenomenon such as depression is the inseparability of the social from the interpersonal, and therefore the 'impersonal' from the 'personal' relations with others. Noting this interconnectivity, the analysis

M. Mirdamadi, *A Phenomenological Study of Depression in Iran*,
https://doi.org/10.1007/978-3-031-30407-1_5

presented in this and the next chapter offers a way of understanding cultural variations and their role in shaping experiences of depression, whilst demonstrating how the dynamics governing the two spheres of social life shape and influence one another, as contexts where experiences arise and are made sense of.

The importance of relationships with others and the phenomenological significance of these cannot be overstated. How we relate to other conscious beings in the world, both as a collective and as individuals, forms an important part of our being-in-the-world, and provides a background for furthering our self-awareness and self-knowledge. These relationships also have a significant role to play in our emotional consciousness and experiences. Given these manifold influences and the significance of interpersonal relationships, an examination of the changes in the way we encounter and relate to others in depression, as well as the role played by culture in shaping these changes, is crucially important.

In giving an exposition of how these factors shape the overall experience of relating to and being with others in depression, it is important to acknowledge the presence of an interpersonal conflict in every domain of our relationships with others. Due to the existential change one goes through in depression, this inevitable, and ever-present conflict between I and Other is brought to the foreground of consciousness, and as such plays an important role in shaping our interpersonal experiences in depression. Whether we focus on stigmatisations of depression as a sign of not being understood by the broader society and its conceptualisations of depression, or on interpersonal understandings and empathy of individual others, an interpersonal conflict is seen to be at the centre of the breakdown of personal bond with others. Heidegger and Sartre are two phenomenologists who take this interpersonal conflict, manifested in different levels of sociality seriously and incorporate it in their discussions. Heidegger's discussion of 'das Man' and its role in shaping an individual's relationship with her wider community, can illuminate the interpersonal conflict as it arises between one and the society at large. Sartre, in contrast, focuses on the interpersonal, one-to-one encounters and relationships with a particular Other and the inescapable conflict that governs the dynamics of these relationships. Together, by bridging the gap between the social and personal realms of relating to and being with others, the two accounts offer a comprehensive theory of the significance and meaning of being with others. These phenomenological accounts, together with the exposition of cultural factors which create the backdrop to interpersonal experiences in depression, provide a framework for understanding some of the cultural variations in experiences of depression.

The Conflict Between the Individual and Her Society

An aspect of experience of depression often talked about by Iranians is the common misconceptions in society regarding the nature of depression itself, which is manifested in stigmatisation or unfair judgements and expectations directed towards the depressed person. I argue that such misconceptions can be theorised in terms of inauthentic understanding of das Man that create a conflict between a depressed individual and her broader society. Therefore, an exposition of Heidegger's theory of our essentially social mode of being-with and the different manifestations of it is needed in order to give an account of the phenomenological significance of this conflict as manifested in depression.

Heidegger views our being as humans as essentially situated within a social world, such that our modes of being and understandings of ourselves and the world around us are always necessarily shaped and influenced by the social world in which we dwell. We are 'thrown' into a world that is always already there and our mode of being is Dasein: being-there. But the world into which we are thrown is a social one and other people are constitutive parts of this world. As such, our mode of being as Dasein is not a solitary dwelling in a world, but a fundamentally social being: Being-with. For Heidegger, the presence of others is always implied in any action Dasein takes and in anything it encounters. The work that Dasein does is destined for others, the practicality of the tools it uses are defined by others and more importantly, Dasein's understanding and view of itself is dependent on the real or imagined presence of others. Dasein finds or loses itself based upon its understanding of and being with others, in particular, from its realisation of how it is different from others. "[W]hether that difference is merely one that is to be evened out, whether one's own Dasein has lagged behind the Others and wants to catch up in relation to them, or whether one's Dasein already has some priority over them and sets out to keep them suppressed." (BT, 27: 126–127) It is in contrast to others that Dasein finds itself, as an individual Being.

We often perceive these differences either as something to be eliminated altogether, thus seeking conformity with others, or as something to be emphasized and developed, in an attempt to distinguish ourselves from others. In both these cases, one allows one's individuality to be determined by others, resulting in an inauthentic individuality—an individuality that is no longer *mine*. This absence of individuality is characteristic of the average everyday being of Dasein, and of the broader society where Dasein finds itself; what Heidegger calls das Man: "[das Man] is neither a collection of definite others nor a single definite Other; it is not a being or a set of beings to whom mineness belongs, but a free-floating, impersonal construct, a sort of consensual hallucination to which each of us gives up the capacity for genuine self-relation and the leading of an authentically individual life" (Mulhall 1996, pp. 68–69). The norms dictated by one's society and culture, are independent of any individual member of that society or culture, yet they influence the way any single person within that society conducts herself, perceives and understands herself. In other words, in every instance during one's daily life, one is representative of one's society, since one necessarily conforms to the norms and values set and dominated by das Man. Therefore, for Heidegger, the average everyday being of Dasein is inauthentic since it takes the form of das Man, such that one's self is one of das Man's.

This everyday inauthenticity is necessary in Dasein's quest for an authentic self. Thus, the ever-present conflict between an individual and her society is made manifest: Each individual Dasein has to continuously overcome the inauthentic das Man and the societal norms and values set out by it, if she is to find her authenticity. The phenomenological experience of a blockade in one's quest remains a negative, frustrating aspect of one's relationship with das Man. Importantly, however, this conflict reaches beyond one's relationship with das Man and permeates her own sense of self and how she relates to the world in which she dwells. Since Dasein's being is essentially being-with, the presence of others and the role of the society is implied in all aspects of her being. This is seen in how Dasein inhabits, and relates to the world, in virtue of her perceptions of it—what Heidegger calls Being-in. Two elements within Heidegger's exposition of Being-in, namely moods and understanding demonstrate the inescapable presence of das Man and its conflict with Dasein.

Moods are basic to our being in the world. They "make manifest 'how one is, and how one is faring'" (BT, 29: 173), since they open up the world to us as significant and meaningful. Separate from emotions, which have a direct object, and sensations, which carry distinctly bodily feelings, moods lack a distinct object. They rather "colour the way everything appears to the self" (Svenaeus 2014, p. 6). Furthermore, moods do not come from the outside or from the inside, they are rather states into which one is always thrown, slipping from one to another or slipping off into bad ones. They are therefore passive states we find ourselves in, inflecting every aspect of Dasein's relation to the world and the entities in it. As such, we find ourselves there in the world, "always already busy with different things that matter to us, and this 'mattering to' rests on an *attunement*, a mood-quality which the being-in-the-world always already has" (Ibid., p. 7).

Since Dasein's being is essentially being-with, the states Dasein finds itself in, such as moods, not only affect, but are affected by its relations to Others. Dasein's membership of a group can lead to her being "thrown into the mood that grips that group, finding herself immersed in its melancholy or hysteria" (Mulhall 1996, p. 79). An individual's social world, its norms, practices and values, fix the moods in which she is thrown, making manifest the role of das Man in determining an individual's mood. The range of possible moods is itself socially moulded: One is more likely to find herself in a mood of elation in a society that values and encourages happiness and expressions of it, both through the expectations that arise as a result of such a valuation, as well as through seeing the way others *are* in the society.

If Dasein is thrown into the world with a certain attunement, understanding is the mode of Being, characterised by moving forward and confronting one's possibilities, given this thrown-ness into the world.

Understanding, for Heidegger, is the act of projecting oneself onto one or other possibility as defined by the world and its attunement. This projection presupposes a grasp of the world Dasein inhabits: a grasp on the world into which Dasein is thrown, and the moods in which Dasein finds itself, together with the objects around it serve Dasein's self-understanding and finding itself in terms of the possibilities presented to it. In choosing to actualise one possibility over others, Dasein is once again faced with the problem of authenticity. In making such decisions, Dasein can either project itself upon a mode of existence in which to express its individuality, or one where it would fail to do so—either through a misunderstanding of its world and possibilities, or through losing itself in das Man and letting das Man determine its choices. As such, this projective understanding itself can be authentic or inauthentic. But in either case, it is always conditioned by the social and cultural situations in which Dasein dwells.

Recall that in Iranian society and culture feeling and expression of sadness is valued insofar as being good in an eternal fight between Good and Evil is valued. This culture is further strengthened by a state that works to highlight and promote ceremonies and events enabling expressions of these affective states. The pre-existing culture and the dominant governing power in Iran work together to create a social mood of sadness and dysphoria, as a state into which individuals are thrown without any particular one having control over it. This mood, however, creates a backdrop to one's perceptions and colours the way she sees and understands herself and the world within it. Crucially, how one understands the world and herself within it, with the use of such moods has implications for the actions one may choose to take. The space of possibilities offered to one is dependent upon one's grasp on the world and the common values and norms within it. This understanding is dependent on the moods and the society in which one resides, but also the actions one chooses to take are shaped by one's attitudes towards her society: should I take an action that is observed by my social peers as desirable and conforming, or should I choose the one that affirms my individuality? In Iran, increasingly young people choose the latter and go against the dominant mood by publicly expressing feelings of happiness and elation. Needless to say, while the general public may condone these actions, the dominant power setting the norms does not. A well-known example is Pharrell Williams' fans, who were sentenced to lashings in 2014, for publishing videos showing them dancing to the song *Happy* (Kamali Dehghan 2014).

These theoretical concepts help to illuminate experience of depression as situated within a social context. The conflict between one and the society in this case translates to one's striving to affirm and validate her individual experiences within a stigmatising understanding of her condition, which in turn determines her possibilities in encountering depression as an illness. The specific role of cultural concepts in this conflict and the concrete experiences are looked at in the next section.

Misunderstanding as Conflict

A general picture of the social experiences of the individual with depression in Iran can be gained through the first-person accounts published on Facebook. These accounts were written unprompted, and as such, the themes individuals chose to write about can be thought to represent what they take to be some of the most important aspects of their experiences. Perhaps unsurprisingly, given the nature of the Iranian society as a collectivist one, the majority of these accounts are concerned with interpersonal relationships, with a particular emphasis on social understandings and attitudes towards depression. What these accounts indicate is a mismatch between the social understanding of depression, and individual experiences of the illness, experienced as a conflict between one and her society. Such misunderstandings are not limited to an abstract definition of depression, but also have implications for judgements and expectations; what they take to be characteristic symptoms of depression, what an individual in depression looks like, and what it means to be depressed. Consequently, they have an impact on individuals' actions and behaviours in their encounter with depression.

The first theme patients talk about concerns the societal misunderstanding of the nature of depression as an illness. The generally accepted conception of illness, in line with the previously discussed cultural concepts inspired by traditional medicine, seems to be one of purely physical nature with perceivable manifestations. Within this understanding, depression is problematic as it is taken to be a purely mental illness with no such observable manifestations. It is therefore difficult for the general public in Iran to accept that such a condition can be a 'real' illness. It should be noted that when Iranians expect an illness to have physical manifestations what is meant are directly observable symptoms of illness, such as tissue damage, or X-ray images of a broken bone. Those behavioural changes that arise in depression, or other mental illnesses, do not seem to be 'physical manifestations' of the right kind. An example illustrating this conception that gets used frequently by Iranians contrasts depression with 'a broken leg':

FB#4 – Nobody expects someone with a broken leg to go hiking … but the difference is you can *see* a broken leg, but you can't see an ill soul.

FB#13 – There is no shame in breaking your limbs. People seek medical help the first opportunity they get and get treatment … but when it comes to depression or mental illness, a lot of people choose silence or denying that the illness exists.

In Heidegger's characterisation, das Man exists in the mode of inauthentic understanding, and is seen as being representative of the widely held beliefs in a given society and seeking conformity with this society. Noting these characterisations makes it clear that such an understanding of illness as always accompanied by directly observable symptoms, and consequently the understanding of depression as a 'less real' illness in the absence of such symptoms, is characteristic of society's inauthentic understanding. Such an understanding is not matched by the individual experiences and is not compromising towards them and therefore creates a tangible conflict between the society and the depressed patients. Stigmatisations and social judgements made about depressed people burdens them with a sense of shame when talking about their experiences. Those suffering from depression carry the burden of rendering their illness and their experience of it legitimate in the face of a society that fundamentally misunderstands their experience.

One response to this misunderstanding seems to be aimed at challenging the supposedly hard division between physical and mental illnesses. Some patients present the various observable manifestations of depression as being close to physical symptoms. One instance of such a response is talk of 'uncontrollable crying' as the most stated symptom of depression among the Facebook sample:

FB#3 – … I would wake up in the morning and start crying. My friend would find a new job I would cry. Stepping on a snail and crushing it would make me cry. It rained, metro was delayed, ATMs were broken, or any other simple reason would make me cry.
FB#4 – [While depressed] any excuse would make my tears flow….
FB#12 – I was done, the me for whom crying was the hardest thing in the world, would now cry when seeing a tiger who had lost its pups on a nature documentary, my soul was extremely weak, so was my tolerance threshold….
FB#14 – Without wanting to, I would cry, without wanting to.

Crying can be seen as a physical manifestation of a non-physical illness. In a society with a tendency to dismiss mental illness as 'unreal' due to not having physical manifestations, an observable manifestation of it could be hoped to play a legitimising role.[1] Crying is also seen repeatedly in the responses to the questionnaire—about 28% of the respondents talk about crying as one of their symptoms of depression. Offering a characterisation of depression that fits in with the widely held beliefs regarding illness generally, would naturally have the effect of eliminating at least some of the stigmas that arise as a result of such misconceptions.

Crying in this context has another legitimising role, namely that of distinguishing between the pathological depressive mood and the normal state of sadness which is only to be expected. The general attunement towards sadness in Iran, and the positive valuation of it, together with the belief that sadness is a necessary and inescapable part of human life, give rise to the social expectation that every individual should be able to cope with this necessary sadness. As a result of this expectation, there is a

[1] It is worth making a note here on self-harming behaviour as a result of social expectations for an individual to legitimise her illness. There is no data on self-harm as a behaviour among depressed patients in Iran, and studies that do exist on the subject often conflate or equate self-harm and suicide attempts, making it difficult to draw precise conclusions about the matter (e.g. Zarghami and Khalilian 2002; Maghsoudi et al. 2004). Although self-harm has not been a common form of behaviour among Iranians, in recent years, the increase in rates of cutting as a form of self-harm among teenage school girls has been reported, sparking worries and a national discussion, especially on the social pressures on young girls in the country (Ilna News 2017).

negative attitude towards those individuals who complain about the presence of sadness in their lives. These are often viewed as weak individuals incapable of dealing with what is seen as a necessary aspect of life. This view is further applied to those suffering from depression: sadness exists for all and complaints about the hardships of life are a mark of a weak character. Uncontrollable crying in such cases acts as an indicator of a deeper form of sadness than what one is expected to endure, or a different form of sadness altogether, one that goes beyond the general attunement of the world and should be considered pathological.

These points serve to indicate the way in which a conflict between individuals and society, between Dasein and das Man, shapes the behaviours of the individuals. Lack of an authentic understanding of depression in society, or even the perception of such a deficiency, forces those suffering from depression to act in a certain way in order to legitimise their suffering and gain the acceptance they need. This lack of understanding, or perception of it, has far reaching effects that extend beyond the social domain and into personal relationships. However, it is important to note here the fact that the influence of such misunderstandings is not limited to the observable behavioural changes. Rather, there are phenomenologically significant consequences, which shape the way in which patients understand and interpret their experiences. One example of such a consequence is the effect of these social misunderstandings on the space of possibilities presented to an individual in depression.

Ian Hacking has shown that social labels and descriptions influence the space of possibilities of actions presented to an individual. Who we are is defined not only by the actions we take, but the possibilities of actions presented to us, i.e. what we might have done or what we might do. However, this space of possibilities is itself bound to social and cultural descriptions: "What is curious about human action is that by and large what I am deliberately doing depends on the possibilities of description … Hence if new modes of description come into being, new possibilities for action come into being in consequence" (Hacking 2002, p. 108). The social judgments and stigmas, stemming from an inaccurate understanding of depression, have practical implications. Specifically, social judgements have the power to shape possibilities for action, as perceived by depressed patients. It is the interplay between the description a community holds, and the individual experiences within the bounds of that description that is of interest here.

Understanding, for Heidegger, is the mode of moving forward in the world, through having a grasp on the world and the possibilities it presents to Dasein. This mode of understanding and the resulting actions are always socially and culturally determined and the presence of das Man, and in turn the possibility of inauthenticity is always embedded in our actions. This sociocultural nature of the mode of understanding and das Man's contribution to it, can have a significant influence on one's grasp of the world in which she dwells and, consequently, the actions or inactions she chooses to take. This can be seen clearly in the case of Iranian patients struggling to identify and carry out their chosen actions in response to depression.

An instance of this interplay is seen in the case of depressed patients who choose medication as their preferred treatment for depression, but who face judgments in light of this decision. Many of the Facebook posts note that taking medication for depression is looked down upon in the society, and that such attitudes result from the lack of understanding of the nature of depression itself:

FB#8 – [The most difficult thing is] explaining to people, making them understand that the state I'm in is not called laziness and is different from short-term and temporary episodes of depression in others, which comes about after emotional crises and failures in employment and studies, that I am trying to get rid of it and of course it crossed my mind, before it crossed theirs, to do something for myself. That it has nothing to do with inculcation … A pain that others, even those closest and dearest to you enforce on you, because they do not know how to act around you so that you do not endure more pressure. That medication is necessary for depression, just like it is for heart disease and diabetes and migraine, that they'd stop blaming you for taking it and recommending herbal remedies and other alternatives.

If such negative attitudes and judgments towards an individual with depression arise from misconceptions of depression rooted in traditional medicine, then it would not be surprising to see these attitudes extend to the medical treatment of depression as well. As noted in Chap. 2, following traditional Iranian and Islamic medicine, the prevalent conception of illness and disease, is one arising from an imbalance in the body, due to environmental, dietary, or stress-inducing factors. In this conception, therefore, one can rid the body of illness through restoring this balance by natural means. Given these folk understandings, herbal remedies and natural alternatives to pharmaceutical medicine have retained a strong preference among Iranians (Loeffler 2007). Through time, however, the success of pharmaceutical medicine has been accepted for somatic illnesses, such as heart disease and diabetes referred to in the above quote. The effectiveness of these for mental illnesses, however, remains controversial in the eyes of the Iranian public.

If we accept, therefore, that there is a negative attitude in society towards taking medication for depression, such a prevalent attitude could have a significant influence on how individuals seek help for depression and the actions they take in treating it. This is again due to the social nature of the world we live in; social and cultural elements not only influence the way we identify our space of possibilities, but also how we choose to act and actualise these possibilities. Given the cultural values of Iran as a collectivist society, the importance of the shared values held by the society and the influence they have on the life choices of the individual, the saliency of this point in the context of Iran is clear. As such, it is not surprising that in some cases attitudes and judgments regarding medication in treating depression are powerful enough that they result in individuals having an altered space of possibilities of action, which in turn influences their choice in which action to take. Therefore, in this context, within a society that not only views depression as somewhat inferior to other, more 'real' physical illnesses, but also has a history of folk theories of illness and treatment which have a negative view of pharmaceutical drugs, the possibility of action for those inclined to such medication as treatment of depression is compromised:

FB#1 – When my family found out about the medicine, they got really upset, it was hard for them to accept that their daughter took antidepressants and this topic is still unacceptable in today's Iran and most often people label you as a mental patient (*bimār-e ravāni*). I stopped taking the medication … I know I need help but my negative personal experience of seeking help from a psychologist, as well as being mindful of my family, and the negative attitude of the society towards those who take medication, stop me from seeking help from psychiatrists and psychologists.

The altered space of possibilities as a result of sociocultural conceptions and misunderstandings of depression, is not limited to taking medication. Iranian patients often complain about their inability to express themselves and their experiences, due to fear of being judged, labelled, or misunderstood. In a society where expressions of one's emotions is encouraged, and where there is an expectation that others would be able to listen and help an individual suffering from unpleasant experiences, the inability to express experiences of depression can be seen as a direct result of misunderstanding and misconceptions of depression. These common misunderstandings in this case, not only limit one's possibilities of action, but further adds to the suffering of the individual, who feels that she has to endure these experiences alone. In the interpersonal domain, such feelings would further add to the patients' feeling of, and tendency towards isolation, as will be discussed further in the next chapter.

FB#3 – I had doubts about writing about my experiences [of depression]. Not because I'm embarrassed, but because those around me clearly see my confession of being depressed as attempting to look intellectual, they think confessing to being depressed has now become fashionable.

FB#12 – I know that writing [about depression] is not going to be without cost for me, I will certainly be judged, blamed, and even sabotaged by friends and acquaintances, colleagues, and even people whom I don't expect.

#33(M) – [In my relations with others I have] an inability to express words, and [therefore] I suffer internally and am unable to express what must be said.

Without being concerned about the authenticity or inauthenticity of such actions (or inactions) taken in light of the social valuations, what is of importance here is the role played by society in shaping the experience of depression in Iranians. What is striking is a sense of uncertainty and unfamiliarity associated with depression and its experiences and treatments. This sense of uncertainty is accompanied by a tension between what an individual experiences in depression, and what the prevalent ideas of society, think acceptable for any individual in that situation. What is interesting is the fact that such social attitudes have a determining influence on individuals' actions, while at the same time having a colouring influence on the individuals' experiences of depression.

In addition to the phenomenological significance of these influences, the cultural dynamics that contribute to this influence in the case of Iran are worth pointing out. For Iranians, having and maintaining a healthy social presence and relationships are of crucial importance. This cultural emphasis and importance is further reinforced by social mechanisms, since having a well-connected network of friends and acquaintances can define an individual's path in life. This centrality of social relationships in Iranian culture and society has been reaffirmed in some empirical studies on cross-cultural beliefs and attitudes towards one's social standing. For instance, Safdar et al. have shown that "for Iranians, paying attention to one's social network (maintaining harmony within it and being sensitive to its complexity) is a way both of getting things done (and thereby gaining a sense of mastery) and of receiving enough positive reinforcement to feel that life is satisfying" (Safdar et al. 2006, p. 128). Given this strong background and context to the influence of social valuations and understandings, it can be seen that these attitudes and the possibilities of action arising from them, contribute to the 'who' of depressed patients in Iran, and the 'how' of their experiences. The possibilities presented to an individual suffering from depression, are determined by the social descriptions of illness and depression, which are themselves culturally determined. The decision to stop taking medication for depression finds significance when considered within the cultural and social context of the decision and the descriptions and judgments that enforce such decisions. And the significance of feeling unable to share one's experiences of depression, even with those close to one, is seen further when considered against the backdrop of sociocultural norms which attach a considerable importance to social relationships.

These considerations, important as they are in themselves, have further consequences. I would argue that the misunderstandings and misconceptions of depression in Iran, and the attitudes and judgments they give rise to, create and maintain a mood of unhomelikeness in the world for the individual in depression. Arising from a sense of not being understood by others, and contributing to a feeling of lack of empathy, this mood dominates the interpersonal relationships in depression. As such, the mood of unhomelikeness can be thought of as a linking point between interpersonal relationships in the broader society, and those in the personal domain. Before looking at how this mood dominates personal interpersonal relationships in depression in the next chapter, I will give an account of how it arises in the social sphere and 'spills over' to the personal domain of relationships.

Conflict, Empathy, and Unhomelikeness

We are always already situated within a world, with people and other entities within it that are meaningful to us. Since the world and the entities in it find meaning for each individual in a unique way, there is always a way in which I feel at home in the world and attach a mine-ness to this world. However, this familiarity of our world, or the sense of 'homelikeness' of the world, is simultaneously pervaded by a sense of homelessness arising from the realisation that one does not fully know or control the world one inhabits. This is a necessary phenomenon since we are thrown into the world with everything and everyone already in it and our being as Dasein is a being-there-in-the-world that finds its own meaning within the disclosed entities. The disturbance of our sense of being at home in the world is always a possibility, and one instance in which this disturbance can be seen clearly is in anxiety arising as a result of the realisation that whilst being mine, the world does not entirely belong to me, thus realising the limitations of my control and effect over the world in which I live. Fredrik Svenaeus, making use of this notion and realising that this sense of 'unhomelikeness' is a necessary aspect of our understanding of the world and so of ourselves, offers an account of illness characterised by this sense. Despite its necessity for an authentic way of life, Svenaeus argues that if persistent, this sense of unhomelikeness becomes characteristic of illness, one which influences our perception of the world and of ourselves within it. (Svenaeus 2000a, 2000b, 2011).

On this account, illness can be understood as a natural event, as a result of which one feels alienated, from one's body, and from her past and future. This alienation leads to an altered view of oneself as well as the world around, one that no longer has the sense of familiarity it once did, thus transforming the homelikeness of the world into unhomelikeness. Whereas health, as a state of homelike being-in-the-world, is characterised by being balanced and in-tune with the world, illness is the state of being off-balance and alienated from all those once familiar. Thus illness is "a state in which the meaning-structure of one's life is challenged, as one's previous state of health is seen in a different light and one is faced with the possibility of creating a new life-meaning" (Kayali and Iqbal 2013, p. 32). The manifestation of the unhomelike quality of the world is different depending on the nature of the illness, yet what remains common in different cases is a change in the way one relates to the world and to oneself in illness.

One example of this unhomelike being-in-the-world is the altered perception of one's body, in an illness which affects one's physical ability. In a state of health, one is able to perform one's daily task without taking notice of one's body. This is while in illness, one becomes aware of one's body through taking notice of the difficulty with which the previously undemanding tasks are performed. In this awareness one takes notice of the limitations on one's bodily capabilities, which in turn affect the way one perceives of the world around her and the possibilities presented to her. One's previous possibilities are seen as less accessible in light of the illness, and the limitations on what one can or cannot do brings home the fact that one is not in control of her body in ways one had previously taken for granted (e.g. Carel 2016).

In the case of depression, this sense of unhomelikeness can be seen in one's altered perception and understanding of the world and entities within it. In depression, due to the existential change one goes through, one's relation with the world and things in it is transformed: the colourful is now seen as colourless, and the meaningful as meaningless. It is in such a case that one in depression loses one's sense of mine-ness in the world, since the world that was mine no longer is, giving it a quality of unhomelikeness. This feeling inevitably affects one's perceptions of, and relations with other people as well, since one's perception of others and their dwelling in the world is altered. The perception of others as kind and loving is changed to one of hostility and untrustworthiness, and it is in this light that one in depression navigates the world and one's relations with people in the world.

Depression is sometimes described as "a creature invading the self and taking control over it." (Svenaeus 2014, p. 4) The consequence of this apparent loss of self and the taking over of the illness, can be seen in the way in which one's world is coloured by depression itself (or drained of colour as a result of it). This new way of perceiving and apprehending the world, which is not necessarily true to the actual reality of the world, is akin to the mood and attunement into which one is thrown when depressed. The mood in depression colours Dasein's world in a new way: one which introduces a different understanding of the world, things and people within this world, and the possibilities for action presented to one. The sense of unhomelikeness in the world is, therefore, one of the ways in which the presence of this mood is felt.

In Iran, the misunderstandings of depression as an illness and the consequent attitudes and judgments directed to one in depression, which are prevalent in the society, contribute to and exacerbate the sense of unhomelikeness. Because of this prevalent lack of understanding, the individual in depression no longer views her social world and people within it as familiar as they once were, since the possibility of mutual understanding is removed from her space of possibilities, thus the presence of interpersonal conflict as an inevitable and ever-present force governing these relationships is dominant in one's encounters with others. The feeling that others cannot understand one and one's experiences, creates for the individual a sense that others can no longer empathise with one. And further, the feeling that others are unwilling or unable to understand one and one's experiences, exacerbates one's sense of unfamiliarity in the world, strengthening the mood of unhomelikeness already felt in depression.

There is an important linguistic note to be made here, regarding the complaints made by Iranian patients about the misunderstanding of depression, and the link between understanding and empathy in Farsi language. Despite there being a word denoting empathy (*hamdeli*),

Iranians often talk about feeling understood by others when talking about feeling empathised with. Understanding is seen as the necessary step for empathy, so much so that in everyday language, the two are often seen and used as synonymous. In such a case, therefore, the existence of misunderstandings in the society of what depression entails and what the appropriate actions in the face of depression are, create a feeling of not being understood, not being empathised with.

This move between understanding and empathy is crucially important, since it makes clear the experience of individuals that goes beyond the perception of a dominant misunderstanding. The conflict between an individual suffering from depression and the society which misunderstands what depression is, adds to a feeling of unhomelikeness in the world, already present in depression. This loss of homelikeness is seen even more clearly when one considers these misunderstandings, as perceived by depressed patients, as instances of lack of empathy on the part of other people. The inability or unwillingness of other people to empathise with the depressed patient, as a central failing in interpersonal relationships, represents the breaking of the interpersonal bond in depression. This perception, which adds to the feeling of unhomelikeness in depression, underlies further feelings and attitudes that exacerbate the failings in interpersonal relationships with specific others.

The inseparability of the social and personal spheres of interpersonal relationships is demonstrated both through the sociocultural norms governing these relations, as well as the ways in which issues and moods in one sphere spill over to the next. The breakdown of the interpersonal bond in the social setting is brought about through a misunderstanding of depression as an illness which hinders understanding and empathy towards individual experiences of it. Instead, the inauthentic understanding gives rise to stigmas and judgments which shrink the depressed person's space of possibilities and her experience of being-in the world and being-with others. This alteration gives rise to a mood of unhomelikeness, which in turn governs one's relations with concrete others. As I demonstrate in the next chapter, unhomelikeness acts as a backdrop against which personal relationships with others, and the emotional experiences in this domain, find meaning and can be understood.

6

Interpersonal Relationships II: Personal Interpersonal

As seen in the previous chapter, one's relationship with others and its changes in depression form a central part of the overall experience of depression. In the preceding arguments, I demonstrated how in depression the inherent conflict embedded within one's relationship with the society one is part of comes to the foreground of consciousness, influencing one's experiences of these relations. In the case of Iranian patients, this conflict can be seen as a form of misunderstanding on the part of the society, of what depression is and how it might be dealt with. In the context of the Iranian linguistic and cultural understanding of empathy, this misunderstanding tends to be interpreted and experienced by depressed people as a lack of empathy on the part of the larger society. This feeling of lack of empathy, in turn, exacerbates the sense of unhomelikeness, as the dominant attunement in depression.

The feelings of empathy, or lack thereof, form the basis of the emotional difficulties felt in depression in relation to others. This principal importance of feelings of empathy, or more accurately, feeling empathised *with,* is seen through the fact that its presence or absence can have crucial implications for interpersonal experiences, including those that are often impaired in the course of depression. In giving an account of what empathy is, Ratcliffe argues that underlying the ability to empathise, is

M. Mirdamadi, *A Phenomenological Study of Depression in Iran*,
https://doi.org/10.1007/978-3-031-30407-1_6

having "a kind of 'openness' to experiential differences" (Ratcliffe 2015, p. 238). It is not the case that in order to empathise, one would necessarily have to experience what another person is experiencing, i.e. moving from the second-person to the first-person in access to a certain experience, giving rise to a "phenomenological isomorphism between the two parties" (ibid., p. 239), as is suggested in other theories of empathy.[1] Rather, what is important is to establish a connection through understanding, whilst acknowledging the phenomenological differences between experiences. This 'openness to difference' in experiences, would be manifested in one's manner in relation to the person having the experience, in the form of curiosity to understand, for example in asking certain questions (or not asking others), being attentive to the Other's needs, etc. Although it is noted that acknowledgment of the phenomenological differences in experience requires some grasp of the other person's experiences, Ratcliffe maintains that "this can remain vague, ambiguous, indeterminate, without amounting to a failure of empathy" (Ratcliffe 2015, p. 239).

Empathy is therefore an attitude towards the experiences of another person. An attitude which seeks to understand and comprehend these experiences as had by the Other, by means of caring, attentiveness, and curiosity. Feeling empathised *with*, therefore, would mean the recognition of this attitude in the Other. This recognition requires an ability to 'connect' with other people, and it is this ability which, because of the existential change one goes through in depression, and as a result of the mood of unhomelikeness dominant in depression, is impaired; the very possibility of attaining and maintaining this interpersonal connection is lost in depression. As a result, therefore, a depressed person is unable to identify in others the empathetic attitudes directed towards her, giving rise to the central feeling of not being empathised with, or not being understood. Such feelings are in turn exacerbated by the continual misunderstanding of depression and the misguided conceptualisations prevalent in the society. This prevalence creates a presumption against which the interpersonal experiences of empathy find meaning.

---

[1] See for instance empathy as simulation in Stueber 2006; Goldman 2006; and mirror or reconstructive empathy in Goldman 2011; De Vignemont 2010.

In this regard, therefore, empathy presents a linking point between the social and the interpersonal problems seen in depression. For the depressed person, the lack of understanding in the social domain creates the expectation of receiving the same behaviour in the interpersonal domain. This loop then carries within it feelings of unhomelikeness as the dominant mood colouring the experiences of interpersonal relationships.

#15(F) – I felt like they didn't understand me/empathize with me.
#6(F) – When I'm depressed, I feel like I don't have an emotional connection with anyone. Nobody can be helpful with their presence.
#2(M) – I feel like they do not have the capability (*tavānāyi*) to understand/empathise at all.

The importance of the recognition of empathy as a linking point between the social and the personal is seen in the emotional experiences and difficulties between individuals and the Other, which arise because of the perceived lack of empathy on the part of others. This perception, together with the realisation and the expectation that one's encounter with the Other, would be similar or representative of one's encounter with others in the society, give rise to emotional experiences as manifestations of the breaking of interpersonal bond, which are culturally and phenomenologically significant.

One of the striking differences between the experiences of Iranian patients and those from the UK, is indeed in the manifestation of the breaking of the interpersonal bond in depression. Most notably, whilst those in the UK complain of feeling lonely in depression, as a result of their inability to connect with other people, Iranians talk about wanting to isolate themselves and 'escape' from other people. This difference points to a conflict in interpersonal relationships made manifest in depression among Iranian patients: It is not the case that people feel unable to connect with other people, but rather that the very desire to do so is lost in depression, and replaced with the desire to seek solitude. This difference and its phenomenological significance is tied to that of the importance of empathy in depression and the emotional responses to the perceived lack of empathy and understanding, as the basis of one's relationship with particular Others.

Relating to Others as Persons

While Heidegger's account of Dasein and das Man is useful in accounting for the dynamics of the relationship between the individual and the society, Sartre's account offers an insight into the interpersonal domain of relationships. At the heart of both of these accounts lies an inevitable conflict, one which for Heidegger arises from the inauthenticity of das Man presenting difficulty for Dasein's quest of authenticity. For Sartre, however, this conflict is much more deeply placed, arising from the conflicting nature between the way an individual sees herself and the way the Other sees her.

A detailed account of the nature of our being is no doubt beyond the scope of this work, however, without diverging from the subject matter, a few observations, made by Sartre, about the nature of our being, illuminate the matter at hand. Sartre observes that the fundamental element in our human consciousness is intentionality—the fact that our consciousness is first and foremost directed outwards and is consciousness *of* something, out there in the world. It follows from this characterisation that our conception of ourselves, the way we see ourselves in the world is fundamentally as subject: my being for my solitary self is one of a self-aware conscious subject. With intentional consciousness as the defining feature of our being, we are subjects with the ability to take things out there in the world as objects of our consciousness. In our awareness of ourselves and the world, therefore, we are conscious subjects aware of other things that comprise our sense of the world in which we dwell, and these other things are always taken as objects of our consciousness, i.e. as things that we are consciously aware *of*. It is this conception of oneself as inherently a subject, which is fundamentally transformed in one's encounter with the Other.

In the presence of the Other, and through the Other's look, my being as a subject is transformed to one of object. This is since, through the recognition of the Other as a conscious being such as myself, I realise the possibility that as a subject, the Other can take me as the object of his consciousness. This recognition of the Other as a person like myself, Sartre claims, comes from certain emotions that I can only feel in the presence of the Other, such as shame and guilt. The very existence of these emotions, the very possibility of feeling these emotions, makes evident the essence of the Other as a person for whose consciousness I can be an object. In such a situation, I realise that the Other *can see me,* and this being seen by the Other, reveals me to myself anew. I now see myself through the eyes of the Other, as I *appear* to the Other, as an object, and through the judgements that the Other can pass on me. "By the mere appearance of the Other, I am put in the position of passing judgement on myself as an object, for it is as an object that I appear to the Other" (Sartre 2003, p. 246).

The presence of others opens up new possibilities for me. Possibilities which rely on the recognition of others as persons, and which include those of meaning-making, the feeling of certain emotions, and understanding of oneself and the world in which one dwells. In Sartre's terminology, in the presence of the Other, my Being for myself—being-for-itself—is transformed into the mode of being of things—being-in-itself—, in the eyes of the Other. And this new mode of being found only in the presence of others, bears no resemblance to what I know myself to be: "I am unable to bring about any relation between what I am in the intimacy of the For-itself, without distance, without recoil, without perspective, and this unjustifiable being-in-itself which I am for the Other" (ibid.). This transformation is crucial for me to realise my being fully, since it makes possible a more complete knowledge of myself, and the feeling of certain emotions, which exist only in the presence of the Other. It is because of this crucial transformation and the new possibilities brought about by it, that Sartre (much like Heidegger), argues that our being as humans is essentially social; it is through our relationships with others that our being is made complete. Sartre argues "I need the Other in order to realize fully all the structures of my being" (ibid.). And it is thus that our being, as a For-itself, is inherently, and essentially, a being-for-others.

This transformation, however, despite opening up new possibilities for one's being, also gives rise to conflicts with the Other. This conflict arises due to the unfamiliar nature of myself in the face of the Other: the Other forces me to see myself in a new way, one which bears no resemblance to the image I hold of myself, i.e. as a subject with certain characteristics.

This objectification of my being by the Other is naturally met with fierce resistance and leads to an unresolvable conflict in which both I and the Other attempt to establish our subject-ness by escaping the inevitable objectification of the other. This struggle is seen in various modes of one's relationship with the Other. From loving to hateful to indifferent, at the heart of all kinds of relationships remains an unresolvable and necessary conflict. This is since in all instances, different in appearance as they might be, the struggle to save one's subjectivity from the look of the Other will be present. "Everything which may be said of me in relations with the Other applies to him as well. While I attempt to free myself from the hold of the Other, the Other is trying to free himself from mine, while I seek to enslave the Other, the Other seeks to enslave me. We are by no means dealing with unilateral relations with an object-in-itself, but with reciprocal and moving relations" (Sartre 2003, p. 386).

However, it is because of this conflict, this constant objectification of myself by the Other, that the possibility of experiencing emotions such as guilt and shame are created. This possibility is not only important for a moral way of being, but is also crucial in one's understanding of oneself. As such, the fact that such emotions are made possible and find meaning in the presence of the Other, makes clear the importance of interpersonal relationships in our emotional lives, despite the existence of an ever-present and unresolvable conflict. Such emotions are made possible because of, rather than despite, the existence of this conflict. It is through interacting with others, and therefore being taken as object of the Other's consciousness, that one sees an image of oneself that might otherwise remain concealed from one's consciousness and therefore experiences. It is not only that through the judgement of others one becomes able to articulate a certain experience or emotion that one was already feeling. Rather, the emotional experiences themselves are brought about through the interaction with others and through the judgements made by others about one. As such, accounting for emotional experiences of depression requires a framework for understanding emotions, in addition to an account of relating to Others. Sartre's theory of emotions together with his account of interpersonal conflict offer the tools for analysing and understanding the Iranian emotional experiences in personal relationships.

Sartre's Phenomenological Theory of Emotions

Sartre's phenomenological account of emotions can be viewed as an attempt at situating emotions within the world one dwells in, since "the notions of the world and of 'human-reality' are inseparable" (Sartre 1962, p. 18). In *Sketch for a Theory of the Emotions* (1962), Sartre situates his account against those from the psychological and Jamesian approaches, which, emphasising the embodied nature of emotions, did not sit neatly within Sartre's existentialist outlook. Instead, Sartre wants to claim emotions to be "an organized form of human existence" (1962, p. 28), a way of acting upon the world highlighted by the 'transformative power' he attaches to emotions.

Aspects of Sartre's theory of emotions continue to be relevant in ongoing debates around the nature of emotions—for instance those that associate emotions with different kinds of mental representations (e.g. Solomon (1992), Nussbaum (2001)); those positing intentionality as a defining feature of emotions (e.g. Goldie 2002); or those emphasising the perceptual nature and basis of emotions (e.g. Prinz (2006)). Yet the account has also been subject to substantial criticisms, particularly those showing the account's shortcomings in providing a general theory of emotions. Instead, it is seen as concerned solely with certain types of emotions considered 'malformed' (Wollheim 1999), 'irrational' (Solomon 2006) or 'distorted or misrepresented' (Richmond 2011). An extended discussion of the merits of Sartre's theory is beyond the scope of this work, yet it should be noted that the discussion of this theory here is not an endorsement of all aspects of it as a general theory of emotions. Instead, I think Sartre's theory of emotions, insofar as it aims to show emotion "possesses a signification of its own" (Sartre 1962, p. 92), offers insight into the *function* of certain emotions in depression. In particular, when understood against the dominant mood of unhomelikeness and the centrality of the interpersonal conflict in depression, Sartre's account can illuminate aspects of emotional experiences in depression arising from the breaking of the interpersonal bond.

On Sartre's account, emotional experiences arise from a synthesis of perception and imagination. One *perceives* the world as limiting and attempts to act upon the world by transforming the possibilities of the world through an act of imagination manifested in emotional reaction to the world. A key component of the function of emotions for Sartre is their transformative power—since in their presence we see the world in a new way and are therefore presented with different possibilities that this new world offers. This transformative nature of emotions is rooted in imaginative consciousness (Sartre 2004) and is viewed as a distinctive feature of emotions. In confronting the limitations of the world one inhabits, perceived as "ruled by deterministic processes" (Sartre 1962, p. 63), one imposes a 'magical quality' onto the world through emotional imagination. And it is thus that for Sartre, "Emotion is a sign of the conscious interpretation man puts on his experience" (Fell 1965, p. 51).

> When the paths before us become too difficult, or when we cannot see our way, we can no longer put up with such an exacting and difficult world. All ways are barred and nevertheless we must act. So then we try to change the world; that is, to live as though the relations between things and their potentialities were not governed by deterministic processes but by magic. (Sartre 1962, p. 63)

Sartre famously uses the example of unripe grapes to demonstrate his case. I reach to pluck a bunch of grapes, but am unable to do so as they are beyond my reach. In response, "I shrug my shoulders, muttering: 'they are too green'" (Sartre 1962, p. 65). Sartre argues that conferring the quality of being 'too green' on the grapes, acts as a substitute for the act which I intended or desired, but was not able to complete. In other words, the attractive quality by which they were presented to me—as 'ready for gathering' as Sartre puts it—, becomes intolerable when the possibility presented to me cannot be actualised. The tension created as a result of this inability to actualise a possibility is resolved when I confer a new quality onto the grapes; i.e. their being 'too green'. Now of course, one cannot confer this new quality chemically, but rather through "putting on the behaviour of disrelish" (ibid., p. 66). I confer the quality onto the grapes 'magically', and it is thus that emotions come about: "In this case the comedy is only half sincere. But let the situation be more critical; let the incantatory behaviour be maintained in all seriousness: and there you have emotion" (ibid.).

What is important for the purposes of our discussion, is that on this account, emotions are like other acts of consciousness: purposive; a way of acting on the world. What Sartre means by an "act of magic" in this case, which underlie the transformative power of emotions, is "act of imagination" (Sartre 2004). The transformation of one's perception of the world, from a deterministic and pragmatic one, into a magical, or imaginative one, enables one to see new possibilities, new ways for apprehending and acting in the world. This is since, in imaginative transformation, the perceived object is transformed so as to conform to our desires directed to the object, it is in this sense that *our feelings remake the object in imagination*. Through this remaking of the object of our emotional consciousness new possibilities arise: the deterministic nature of the environment no longer presents itself as a limiting condition, since the new quality projected onto the world (or a certain object within the world), presents to one's consciousness a new way of apprehending the world. This new apprehension, then, presents new potentialities, new possibilities, and new ways to act upon one's desires, by directing one's emotional consciousness to the world.

Taking this Sartrean framework for analysis, delineating both the nature of relating to others as individuals, and the function of emotions particularly in cases of perceived limitations on space of possibilities, emotional experiences in depression can be accounted for. Arising from the breaking of the interpersonal bond and highlighting the ever-present interpersonal conflict, such experiences can be understood against the 'frustrating' conditions of limitation and lack of empathy that merit strong emotional reactions (Elpidorou 2017).

Emotional Experiences in Depression Among Iranians

If the attunement of unhomelikeness and the perceived lack of empathy among depressed patients is the background of relations with others, emotional experiences are the manifestation of the breaking of interpersonal bond in depression. The perceived lack of empathy brings the conflict between I and the Other to the foreground of consciousness and experiences and results in the experience of certain emotions which dominate Iranians' experience of depression. Thus, in addition to feelings of lack of empathy and loss of interpersonal connection, Iranians often talk about having negative emotions towards others, or being on the receiving end of negative emotions. These emotional experiences, in addition to being important in themselves, give rise to specific experiences and behaviours, an account of which would be incomplete without considering the role of the underlying emotions.

As shown in Sartre's account of emotions, perception and imagination are key elements in emotions. In the case of depression, the perceiving act, is one of lack of empathy on the part of others, the inability to recognise the empathetic attitude in others. In forming a reaction to this perception, one's imagination and apprehension of this perception which are projected upon the world in emotions, are governed by the dominant mood of unhomelikeness in depression and define the space of possibilities and one's view of others and the world. It is in this dynamic that one fails to connect with other people: "a kind of interpersonal connection that many of us take for granted seems *impossible*, absent from the world" (Ratcliffe 2015, p. 218). Instead, what is highlighted in this dynamic, is the constant and ever-present conflict between one and Others. As such, this dynamic offers a way of understanding the way in which the interpersonal bond breaks down in depression; rather than considered in isolation, this breakdown finds meaning when considered in its entirety with different connected elements, emotional, behavioural, and cognitive alike. Throughout the following account, it should be borne in mind that the attunement of unhomelikeness dominates the way one thinks and apprehends one's perceptions of others.

#6(F) – I see what they do and their behaviours in a pessimistic/negative way. The routine (*roozmarreh*) behaviour of, for example, my parents become agitating (*asabi*) to me.

This way of seeing others is key in the analysis, since it is against this background that emotions come about, and it is through this background that the possibility of apprehension in a positive way is removed.

Negative Emotions

Although problems caused by misunderstandings of depression are prevalent in both social and interpersonal domains, there is a subtle difference between the manifestations of this misunderstanding in the two domains. Due to the intimate nature of interpersonal relationships, the misunderstanding of depression in this domain is manifested, not through general judgments and misunderstandings, but rather through various expectations of certain behaviours and explanations. Patients often complain of other people's inability to understand their illness experiences, which in turn demands explanations that they are not always equipped to give.

#1(F) – I'm not in the mood for having contact [with others] … everyone wants to know why I'm not the happy and smiling person I used to be and this makes me more isolated.
#2(M) – The most important thing I can think of [is] the explanation as to why I sleep so much, why I cannot work, why I don't take part in family activities and why I have become so weak/powerless (*nā-tavān*) without a physical problem.
#33(M) – [Others annoyed me] by saying 'you don't feel well, why are you like this, you look unwell, the way you speak is different'.

What is noteworthy here is the fact that these expectations arise from the social misunderstandings and misconceptions of depression itself. It is not the symptoms themselves, such as lack of energy and fatigue, that are questioned, but rather the presence of these symptoms in the absence of a physical illness. Once again, the patients are seen to be asked to legitimise their illness in a way so as to conform to the pre-existing assumptions and conceptualisations of what constitutes an illness.

However, there is an undeniable difference between the reactions to such judgments and expectations in the interpersonal domain, compared to the social sphere, namely the perceived personal nature of these judgements. It can be clearly seen from the responses from patients, that the lack of understanding and empathy, perceived in the interpersonal domain, does not concern depression itself, or one's experiences. Rather, patients feel that they themselves are not being understood, and other people do not have the capacity to understand them, as a person.

#17(F) – I feel like others also are not in the mood for [dealing/being with] me and … I feel like they don't understand/empathise with me.
#14(F) – I felt like they didn't understand/empathise with me.

This personal nature of the perceived judgment can be interpreted phenomenologically as the feeling of the Others passing judgements as to *the kind of person that I am*. As such, distinct from the specific experiences and the underlying causes, such a perception of the attitudes taken towards one can be interpreted as an unkind judgment on one's very way of being, and thus can be an instance of the conflict that Sartre construes between the self and the Other. Once construed in this way, the attitudes and emotions that one takes as reactions towards the Other can be made sense of. However, it is not only on the grounds of the perception that others are not able to, or willing to understand one that these reactionary attitudes arise.

The perception that those close to one do not have the capability to understand one is formed against the backdrop of the attunement of depression as unhomelikeness. In this sense, then, one sees others as adopting a hostile view towards one. This perception of hostility, as an instance of the breakdown of the interpersonal bond, despite the differences in its manifestations, seems to be a universal part of the experience of depression. "All that others are perceived to offer is a distinctively *personal* form of threat, which might be experienced more specifically as derision, dismissal, ridicule, condemnation, aggression, or shame" (Ratcliffe 2015, p. 220). These various manifestations of this perceived hostility are present among the Iranian patients as well, and they persist even in the absence of others.

#14(F) – My sister didn't apprehend that I had depression, she felt my aim was to get attention from the family.
#25(M) – Others get upset and say that I'm trying to be classy.
#17(F) – I feel like others … also talk behind my back and talk [badly] about me.
#24(M) – My family hates me.
#30(F) – [Others' encounter] has made [my experience] worse – the way they are with me is really bad.

What is clear here, is the perception of a wide range of negative attitudes, judgements and emotions directed to one in depression. This perception brings to the foreground the conflict between the individual and the Other, formed in this case, due to the lack of understanding on the part of others. Despite the fact that these feelings may be merely perceived, coloured by the dominant mood of depression, this perception is a necessary step for the creation of other emotions. The perception of the world being a certain way, with one's possibilities limited as a result of this, motivates the creation of reactionary emotions, which take the form of negative emotions towards others. These negative emotions can be accounted for through two separate but linked considerations. The first is the already mentioned theory of emotions: as a result of the perception of negative attitudes and judgements directed towards one, and in the background of the mood of unhomelikeness which dominates one's thoughts and outlook to the world, one comes to feel certain negative emotions towards others. Secondly, in the context of the conflict between one and the Other, the perception that the Other is passing judgements on one and sees one in light of these judgements, is experienced as objectification by the Other. As seen earlier, when faced with such feelings, one inevitably moves to re-establish one's subjectivity by taking the Other as the object of one's consciousness and one way of doing this is through one's emotional consciousness towards the Other.

#21(F) – I dislike everyone and nothing seems good to me. I feel hatred towards my children and family and want to escape from them.
#7(F) – Sometimes in depressive periods I would really really hate my father.
#31(F) – I dislike them all [family and friends].
#28(F) – My brain didn't believe what anyone was saying, like a person who hears something from one ear and it goes out from the other ear [Persian expression].

It is important to recall here the importance of such emotions, as instances of action taken by individuals in depression, but also as representative of their experiences and interpretation of their perception of the world around them. The feeling of hatred towards others, as well as being seen as a reaction to the perceived negative attitudes and emotions towards the individual, are representative of the way one interprets one's position among others in the world. As such these emotions are also informative of the way one sees the world more generally. The feeling of being stuck and the general sense of dissatisfaction with life (as seen in Chap. 4) are echoed in the emotions towards others. Sartre acknowledges this interconnectivity of one's emotional consciousness and sees this connectivity as an important pillar of emotional experiences as significative of the one's being more generally. "The impossibility of finding a solution to the problem is apprehended objectively, as a quality of the world. This serves to motivate the new unreflective consciousness which now grasps the world differently, under a new aspect, and imposes new behaviour – through which that aspect is grasped …" (Sartre 1962, pp. 64–65). It is in this new apprehension of the world that another variation in manifestations and experiences of depression between Iran and the UK finds meanings and significance.

Aggression and Guilt

Feelings of guilt and shame are associated with being negatively evaluated, by the self or the Other respectively, as a result of one failing to meet certain norms and standards of what is considered right or appropriate.

This is why these feelings are regarded as 'moral' emotions (Wong and Tsai 2007). Shame and guilt are also instances of 'self-conscious' emotions, "because they require a concept of the self, or an ability to see the self as an object of evaluation" (ibid., p. 210). This concept of the self plays a central role in accounting for a striking difference between manifestations of depression in Iran and the UK, namely the absence of feelings of guilt among Iranian patients, and instead the presence of aggressive behaviour towards others.

As has been noted, an important cultural difference between Iran and the UK, crucial in the analysis of interpersonal problems, is the way in which social relationships are construed within the culture. As a collectivist society, Iranian culture places heavy emphasis on shaping and maintaining social relationships, where the aims and goals of the individual are thought to have a lower priority than those of the collective group. This is in contrast to the individualistic nature of the UK society, in which the aims of the individual take precedence over the goals of the group. One important point arising from this structural difference, is one to do with the construction of the concept of self. "Individualistic societies are best characterized by their conception of an *independent self* that is bounded, unique, and generally autonomous … social behaviour is generally judged to be driven from within and attributed to an individual's internal attributes" (Goetz and Keltner 2007, p. 158). This is in contrast to (mostly) non-Western, collectivist cultures, where "an *interdependent self* is seen as part of an encompassing social relationship, recognizing that one's 'self' is determined by one's relationship with others and the group" (ibid.). Individuals in collectivist societies, further, tend to attribute the causes of events in their lives to external sources, events, or people, as seen in the responses of depressed patients as well, who attribute the cause of their depression to a source independent of themselves (see Chap. 2). In other words, in explaining events in their lives, individuals from collectivist societies are more likely to hold external factors, including other people as responsible.

Iranians often do favours for one another, friends and strangers alike, without being asked to do so, for example putting up banners and streetlights to welcome a neighbour from a long journey, or congratulating them on an achievement. The expectation that others will always be there for one when one is in need, and will care for one, is central in the normal day to day relations with others. However, the perception of lack of empathy on the part of others, as seen in depression, can be thought of as an instance where this expectation is not met. As a result, Iranian depressed patients feel a sense of abandonment by others, as well as disappointment that their expectations are not met. Feelings of abandonment and disappointment are seen in the complaints of patients regarding the way others react to their depression experiences and form the basis of holding others—at least in part—responsible for the pain that they go through. Such feelings are in direct contrast to the feelings of patients in the UK. For instance, whilst those in the UK talk about feeling as if they have become a burden on Others, in Iran patients talk about Others being bored and tired with their depression, and therefore adopt negative attitudes towards them. In other words, whilst for those in the UK, feelings of resentment and responsibility are turned inwards towards oneself, in Iran such feelings are turned outwards towards Others.

#27(F) – I felt that others were also tired of my depression.
#17(F) – Others get bored with my depression and always question/annoy me.

Such way of reasoning, as a point of difference between patients in Iran and the UK, can in part explain the absence of guilt and presence of aggression among Iranian patients. Criticism and dissatisfaction directed towards oneself is more likely to translate into feelings of guilt and wrongdoing. This is while, criticism directed outwards to Others motivates an outward reaction in the form of aggressive behaviour. Furthermore, as seen in Chap. 4, a large part of the experience of depression for Iranians is centred around a feeling of dissatisfaction with the world and the people in it. While the object of one's feeling of dissatisfaction with life and the world may remain vague, when such feelings are directed towards other people, the object of the feeling is very much accessible.

Another factor that plays an important role in bringing about aggression, has to do with the interpersonal conflict that is brought to the foreground of consciousness in depression. As noted above, part of what the interpersonal experience in depression involves is that depressed people tend to feel that Others are hostile towards them, as seen in the perception of negative emotions directed towards one which elicit an affective response. In such cases, where one feels that her sense of self is being threatened by the negative valuations and judgments, and especially where one does not see oneself as responsible and is thus resistant to feelings of guilt, aggression and aggressive behaviours are more likely to come about (e.g. Stuewig and Tangney 2007). The feeling of being misunderstood, receiving judgments which bring into question the 'reality' of one's illness and one's motivations for 'appearing ill', can be perceived as an attack on one's sense of self, which warrants reactions of anger and aggression. As seen in Sartre's characterisation of the interpersonal conflict, in relations with the Other one is constantly made to reassert oneself as a subject, in response to feeling threatened by the Other's objectification of oneself. Against the backdrop of the breaking of the interpersonal bond, one in which lack of understanding, negativity and hostility define one's encounter with the Other, aggressive behaviour could be thought of as a strong attempt to reassert oneself in response to the perceived attacks of the Other.

#20(F) – I become aggressive, I don't answer the phone and am not in the mood for [being with] others, or I tell them not to call me or to stay away from me.
#6(F) – I get aggressive. I don't have the tolerance for the simplest disagreements or arguments.
#7(F) – I'm either completely defeated (*maghloob*), or angry and aggressive, or quiet (*sāket*) and stagnant/static (*rāked*).
#25(M) – I would get angry really quickly and easily … I can't be kind to my children, I can't go to my shop and I always want to commit suicide or kill the one who has betrayed me.

Due to the variety and interconnectivity of the different elements at play here, it is difficult to single-out one element as the cause of the presence of aggressive behaviour in Iran and its absence in the UK. However, what should be clear from the analysis here is that a multiplicity of cultural norms and expectations and the severity of problems in the interpersonal and social domains in depression, and the range of emotions in reaction to these problems together give a convincing picture of the cross-cultural difference. A plausible claim is that the totality of these problems can be seen in the frame of the interpersonal conflict, one that is exacerbated in depression, and from which the individual attempts to escape, when faced with its severity and the impossibility of finding a resolution. This conflict is the 'problem', as Sartre argues, that motivates one's imagination to conceive of different emotional and behavioural reactions. And as one perceives the conflict as more difficult to resolve, so the reactions to resolve it grow in intensity. In the social domain the conflict between one and the society alters the patients' space of possibilities of action, for instance in the case of taking medication and expressing one's experiences. The same misunderstandings and the resultant perception of lack of empathy on the part of Others, create the conflict in interpersonal relations. Importantly, in the case of Iran, due to the strong entanglement between individuals, as well as between the individual and the social groups and society, where the lines between private and public life, between one and the Other, are blurred, one is neither able to resolve this conflict, since in light of the depressive mood such a possibility is not even conceived, nor to escape from it. And it is in this dynamic which the most prevalent and talked about difference between the depressed patients in Iran and the UK is seen, namely, voluntary isolation and escape from others.

Isolation

The most notable difference in experiences of interpersonal relationships in depression between Iran and the UK, is in people's solitary tendencies. Ratcliffe shows that those suffering from depression in the UK often talk about a sense of solitude and loneliness, one that goes hand in hand with a sense of estrangement from the world more generally. On Ratcliffe's account, this feeling of loneliness is closely tied with that of lack of empathy and not being understood: "there is a *feeling* that [others] do not understand, which could equally be described as a feeling that they unable to 'relate to' or 'connect with' the depressed person" (Ratcliffe 2015,

p. 202). As such, lack of understanding is construed as evidence of the breakdown of the interpersonal bond, which leads to the depressed person feeling estranged from others, overcome by a sense of loneliness and solitude.

In the case of Iran, however, there is no talk of feeling lonely. Rather, Iranian depressed patients often express a desire to escape from others and to be alone (26% of the sample). Two important notes should be made with regards to this difference. Firstly, that the state of isolation from others is not only not complained about, but represents a desired state of being. Secondly, despite the feeling of lack of understanding present in both contexts, this feeling does not amount to a sense of estrangement from others, i.e. *willing*, but being *unable* to establish an interpersonal connection with others, as it does in the UK. Both of these elements can arguably be accounted for through the interpersonal conflict which dominates one's relationships with others in depression, and the differences in terms of the kind of society and the kind of prevalent norms in which the individuals are thrown.

#15(F) – I was always in a corner not talking to anyone [the phrase is 'being in myself'] … I was hermitic/withdrawn (*goosheh-gir*), avoided gatherings, was not in the mood to be around anyone.
#17(F) – I'm not in the mood to be in social gatherings with friends and prefer more to be withdrawn/hermitic.
#18(M) – [I] go back into my shell and stop interacting with others.
#19(F) – When I'm depressed, I don't want to talk to anyone or go anywhere.
#23(F) – When I'm depressed, I isolate/withdraw myself and become hermitic … I am not really in the mood for them [other people], because I like to be alone when I'm depressed.
#25(M) – I want to be alone and have nobody around me.
#27(F) – I am not even in the mood for myself and I like to be alone … I'm not in the mood for anyone around me … I'm not in the mood to be with others at all and only want to be alone.

In depression, the conflict between one and the Other dominates one's frame of thought and one's relationship with others. The conflict, represented in the endless loop of not understanding, negative attitudes and emotions, and aggression, is seen to be unresolvable. In other words, due to the circle of negative experiences and negative thoughts and attitudes, the very possibility of re-establishing the personal bond, one that is constructive rather than destructive, is removed from one's space of possibilities. In this case, then, the only change in one's behaviour that could result in the reduction of the conflict and the negativity that comes with it, is to remove oneself from social interactions, i.e. to escape from the interpersonal relationships and the conflict that they present.

The emphasis placed on personal relationships in the collectivist culture of Iran underlies the significance of the possibility of escape as the only available option in reducing the anguish of interpersonal relationships in depression. An example of this cultural emphasis is the fact that despite certain changes, living alone remains an unacceptable way of life for most Iranians. It is generally accepted that the best way of life is one that puts family at the centre, and this means that the majority of people live with family members, either the one they were born into, or the one they married into. In contrast, a life separate from family is seen as a flawed and incomplete way of life. Ultimately, norms such as this mean that the only way one could have a personal space to oneself, is by retracting from the everyday way of life, which is defined by the constant presence of, and contact with other people. In such a scenario, one does not *feel* alone, as there is always an Other present and as has been seen, this presence often brings with it feelings of conflict. This ever-present nature of the interpersonal conflict forces one to try and retract oneself from the social situations.

Furthermore, the cultural norms of interacting with others and being a certain way in the presence of others could be seen as adding more pressure on the depressed patients and in turn exacerbate the feelings of conflict in depression. An example of such expectations, which is especially strong in the case of women, is that one is expected to visit one's parents regularly, or be hospitable to anyone who comes to visit one, whether invited or not. Particularly in rural areas, where more traditional ways of life and roles are in place, women may be the ones in charge of taking care of the family and the house. Such gender roles help make sense of the fact that women are often the ones who complain of being unable to be hospitable, kind to their children, and visiting family members. About a third of all the female respondents express such complaints, compared to only one male respondent who complained of inability to care for his children well. Similarly, although most respondents complain of the disruption depression causes to their work routine, women are more likely to specifically talk about housework and caring duties, compared to men who complain of having to cancel business dealings, or being otherwise unable to work outside of the house. The fact that depressed patients talk about not being able to act as social norms dictate, can be seen both as a way of talking of an inability in illness to legitimise the suffering they go through, as well as a source of pressure that makes the case for escaping from the social interactions ever so stronger.

#28(F) – [I am] hermitic/withdrawn, I stay away from social situations … in most cases I isolate myself and don't want to go see anyone, or let any visitors to come and see me … I don't take part in any social gatherings, be it a funeral/mourning or weddings, and I'm not in the mood for [being around] my children and am mostly just with myself and isolated.

#21(F) – I isolate myself and really don't like to interact with anyone, or if anyone comes to visit me I don't feel like being hospitable.

#28(F) – I stay away from others and stay at home alone and don't have any relation with others, I don't even go to my father's house.

In discussing the experience of the break in interpersonal bond in depression, two different but intimately linked elements ought to be acknowledged. In the first instance, there are universal experiences of being with and relating to others which are made sense of through the universal structures of our consciousness, as laid out by phenomenological considerations. In this sense, the accounts offered by Sartre and Heidegger help to understand the presence of an ever-present conflict between I and others in both social and interpersonal domains that come to the foreground of consciousness and experiences in depression. The second element is the sociocultural norms and customs which shape the manifestations and experience of this breakage in interpersonal bond and influence the emotional and behavioural responses to it. What the preceding account once again demonstrates, is the interplay between these considerations and the incompleteness of one without the other. Furthermore, it is through acknowledging this interplay that the two domains of interpersonal relationships, the personal and the impersonal, can be viewed and analysed together. Sociocultural conceptions that are prevalent in society influence one's expectations and modes of conduct in personal encounters with Others, while the dominant mood in one sphere carries through to the other, forming the background against which interpersonal experiences are shaped. Viewed in this way, cultural variations between experiences and manifestations of depressive experiences in the social domain can be accounted for.

7

The Body in Depression

Somatisation of depression is a feature often talked about in cross-cultural studies of depression. One prevalent claim is that patients in non-Western cultures tend to talk more about physical symptoms in depression, as compared to those from Western cultures who predominantly complain of psychological and emotional difficulties (e.g. Kleinman 1977; Tseng 1975). Various arguments and reasons for this phenomenon have been suggested. On the one hand there has been the suggestion that people from non-Western countries, as well as those from lower socioeconomic backgrounds are less able or less willing to express psychological and emotional distress (Crandell and Dohrenwend 1967; Kleinman 1982), while others have suggested that patients in Western countries tend to overemphasise the psychological symptoms and underemphasise the physical symptoms that, they too, experience (Ryder et al. 2008; Parker et al. 2001; Kirmayer 2001).

What seems to be agreed is the fact of the presence of somatic symptoms, to different degrees and with varying manifestations across different cultures. Indeed, there are certain physical sensations which are thought to be a universal part of the experience of depression (Haroz et al. 2017), including the sensation of the body as heavy and leaden, and feelings of physical weakness. Even though certain physical symptoms are seen universally, there are differences in the emphasis placed on different somatic symptoms which ought to be accounted for.

M. Mirdamadi, *A Phenomenological Study of Depression in Iran*,
https://doi.org/10.1007/978-3-031-30407-1_7

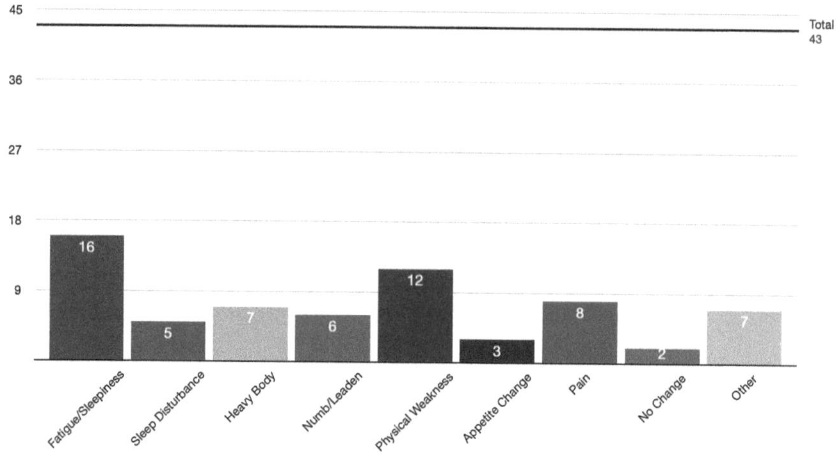

Fig. 7.1 Somatic symptoms complained about by Iranian depressed patients

One of the questions the Iranian sample was asked, concerned somatic symptoms of depression, and Fig. 7.1 represents the different symptoms and their frequency reported in the sample. Here, similar complaints have been grouped together to get a better picture of the frequency of different symptoms. For instance, respondents' complaints of exhaustion and fatigue are often accompanied by complaints of feeling sleepy or 'having a tendency towards sleep'. By grouping these two complaints together, I signify the fact that they often appear together, as well as differentiating this kind of complaint from those related to 'sleep disturbance' where people complain of sleeping excessively or not enough. Similarly, complaints grouped under 'physical weakness' encompass different descriptions of feeling feeble, weak, and lacking in energy. The descriptions of the body, or its perception as heavy, shattered, beaten, or bent are grouped together to signify disturbances to the way the body appears to one, as a limiting force. Lastly, the grouping of feeling numb and leaden together is due to linguistic complexities, since the word used by respondents to describe this state, *kerekh/kerekhti*, can signify both 'numb' and 'leaden' feelings in the body. Symptoms under 'other' represent scattered complaints that are few in number and unrelated to other groups. In this category there are complaints of anxiety and heart palpitations (3), hand trembling (1), sweaty palms (1), and the feeling of body in unrest (1) and an agitated state (1).

Presentation of somatic symptoms and the varying emphases placed on them across cultures, is a multifaceted phenomenon. In its totality, these symptoms form part of the embodied experience of depression which is noteworthy for any phenomenological analysis. However, how this disturbance is experienced, understood and interpreted by the individual and in turn communicated to others, relies heavily on the sociocultural frameworks of understanding. Furthermore, somatisation of mental disorders may, in certain social settings, take on a legitimizing role or act as a tool to escape stigmatisation. Noting this interconnectivity of different factors at play, it is worth clarifying the significance of somatisation of depression in the Iranian context, before sketching the phenomenological importance of the symptoms.

Somatisation of Depression in Iran

The term 'somatisation' has been employed in the literature of mental disorders to denote a variety of phenomena and illness behaviours, which whilst overlapping, are conceptually distinct (Kirmayer and Robbins 1991). There are at least three distinct ways of understanding the term as identified by Simon and others (1999).

In the first understanding, the term highlights presentation with somatic symptoms, such that patients suffering from a psychiatric illness primarily seek help for physical difficulties. In such cases, the somatic symptoms are the primary source of concern for the patient, rather than, for example, any behavioural changes due to the underlying psychiatric illness. The second definition emphasises the association between psychological disorders and medically unexplained somatic symptoms, where psychological distress heightens the perception or the reporting of somatic symptoms, a phenomenon known as somatosensory amplification. Lastly, the third understanding of the term emphasises the lack of expression of psychological symptoms and the substitution of somatic symptoms in their place. On this understanding, linked to the inability to express one's feelings and emotions, somatisation presents "a psychological defence against the awareness or expression of psychological distress" (Simon et al. 1999, p. 1330). An example of this latter form of somatisation is Kleinman's discussion of somatisation of depression in China, where expression of emotions and emotional distress is looked down upon (Kleinman 1982). Kleinman has construed this form of somatisation as an instance of idiom of distress in cultures where psychiatric illnesses carry significant stigma (Kleinman 1977).[1]

Somatisation in Iran can be characterised using the second definition, where somatic symptoms, as the embodied experience of depression, are significant in shaping the overall experience of depression, and should therefore be viewed and accounted for as such. Responses to the questionnaire indicate that despite their presence, somatic symptoms were not the primary reason for depressed patients to seek medical help. These were rather, secondary symptoms accompanying the psychological difficulties, such as feelings of sadness, hopelessness, and suicidal thoughts, which were the patients' primary worry. The emphasis on the emotional and/or psychological symptoms further discounts the notion of somatisation as a masking or substitution of other underlying symptoms. Within Iranian culture emotions and feelings are of central importance in the way one views oneself and relates to other people, and therefore, unlike some other cultures, such as China, expressions of emotional distress are not discouraged or looked down upon.

However, given the previous discussions of misunderstanding and stigmatisation of depression in Iran, the higher emphasis on somatic symptoms can also be attributed to patients' attempts at countering prevalent stigmas. As discussed previously, the stigma attached to depression in Iran is in part due to the cultural way of understanding illness as one which, if not a purely physical entity, has at least some physical manifestations. This understanding of health and illness, traceable to traditional Iranian medicine, partly explains why complaints of somatic symptoms are seen more frequently in Iran compared to the UK. Somatic symptoms in Iran, such as pain, can therefore be seen as a means of escaping stigmatisation and legitimising depression as a 'real' illness (similar to uncontrollable crying seen in Chap. 5). In other words, somatisation of

[1] The notion of idioms of distress will be looked at in more detail in the next chapter.

depression provides a stigma-avoiding strategy in Iran, similar to its role in China, not because of cultural norms against the expression of psychological and emotional difficulties, but due to cultural ways of understanding what constitutes an illness.

When examining first-person accounts of somatisation, however, discerning the intended meaning of the reports and therefore understanding the significance and function of somatisation is not always straightforward. Instead, due to conflation of metaphorical and literal use of language, there are often alternative ways of understanding reports and complaints of somatisation. This is the case, I suggest, with some previous research on somatisation of depression in Iran.

In their research, Byron and Mary-Jo Good report a high prevalence of somatisation of depression among Iranian patients. The most commonly complained about physical symptom is heart distress (*nārāhati-e qalbi*), which they characterise as "a condition associated with physical sensations of heart palpitation, pressure on the chest, and a sensation of the heart being squeezed" (Good et al. 1985, pp. 392–393). Noting that in Iranian popular culture the heart, as well as being a physiological organ, is the core of one's self, they argue that "complaints of heart distress are often associated with feelings of sadness or dysphoria as well as anxiety" (ibid., p. 393). Construing heart distress as an idiom of distress among Iranians, which carries cultural significance, they argue that this symptom ought to be regarded as a somatic framework in which depression and anxiety are often articulated. Good and Good take the expressions of physical distress at face value and therefore offer an understanding based on the literal meaning of the complaints. I would suggest an alternative understanding, whereby expressions of 'heart distress' should rather be understood metaphorically.

Nārāhati-e qalbi is a general phrase, used commonly to the present day to describe various heart diseases, and denotes an exclusively physical illness. It is true that in addition to being a physical organ, the heart is significative of the core of one's self and the source of all emotions and feelings. However, what is lost in translation is which meaning of 'heart' is intended on different occasions where the word is used. Sometimes when patients complain of sensations involving the heart their complaints should be understood literally. For example, in the following remarks made by patients responding to the questionnaire used in this study, what is described is a physical experience that accompanies feelings of anxiety and distress.

#14(F) – [I feel] an inner anxiety that would fill my whole self and I would have heart palpitations.
#2(M) – [I feel] exhaustion and sleepiness. Sometimes accompanied by intense anxiety and heart palpitation.
#38(F) – [I had] heart palpitations, problems breathing, I felt something bad was going to happen to me.

Such experiences are not exclusive to Iranian patients (Sartorius et al. 1996; Lamers et al. 2011) and therefore cannot be thought of as a cultural syndrome.

These descriptions are, furthermore, distinct from ones where talk of a sensation in the heart or another part of the body is used to convey emotional distress. In these latter forms of complaints, the metaphorical use of the word *qalb* (heart), or more commonly *del* (meaning the stomach as a physical part of the body, but also the heart, as the source of one's emotions), for example in the expression of the sensation of one's heart being squeezed, denotes a feeling of sadness and sorrow, often accompanied by tendency to cry and isolate oneself from the world, rather than any physical sensations. The same could be said for the various expressions centred around the heart, most of which express an emotional rather than a physical experience. The conflation of the two very different meanings and employment of the word in everyday language, causes difficulties in discerning the intended meaning of the complaints. I suggest that the fact that such expressions are commonly used in Iran to denote emotional distress, rather than physically felt symptoms, means that such reports cannot be taken literally as describing instances of somatisation.

Byron Good argues that heart distress is a disease category, with various physical sensations such as the pounding, trembling and fluttering of the heart, which are associated with feelings and emotions. This claim further finds support from the fact that people who complain of such sensations attribute the causes to various emotional difficulties, such as sadness, grief, and stress. Therefore, Good argues that heart distress, as an illness, "is perceived as a complex which includes and links together both physical sensations of abnormality in the heart beat, and feelings of anxiety, sadness, and anger" (Good 1976, p. 36). I suggest instead that the various expressions used in describing these 'physical sensations' are used metaphorically and rather than referring to an actual physical difficulty and distress in the heart, are ways of expressing emotional distress. In other words, heart distress is not an illness category which links physical and emotional experiences together, but rather, it represents a way of articulating one's emotional state and the suffering resulting from some of these states, in terms of physical and bodily experiences. The fact that these expressions are linked with physical sensations in the heart should not be taken as evidence that these are somatic symptoms of mental illnesses, but rather, that the place of the heart in the Iranian culture is a fundamental one representing one's emotions and inner state. And as such, the expressions are to be understood as statements regarding one's emotional experience, rather than somatic illness.

An important point to be drawn from this discussion is the fact that often Iranians talk about their emotional experiences using terms denoting physical parts of the body. Whilst some of these articulations can be phenomenologically interesting and significant, such as the feeling of being 'droopy' or 'bent' which express a state of one's being through inducing a physical image of the state of body, a knowledge of the culture, and cultural ways of employing language and expressions is required in order to offer an account reflecting the experiences of those uttering the expressions. Part of the reason why Iranians talk about their emotional experiences in terms of physical sensations can once again be traced to theories in traditional medicine, where physical and psychological experiences are seen as inseparable, each influencing the other. An overview of the ways in which the physical and psychological are tied together in traditional medicine, can demonstrate the cultural tendency towards using physical body parts to talk of emotional experiences, in turn offering insight into a more culturally nuanced analysis of somatisation.

Cultural Conceptions and Somatisation

As noted earlier, the Iranian conceptualisation of depression is in part informed by the conceptions of health and illness theorised in traditional Iranian and Islamic medicine. In this characterisation, psychological and physical ailments are dependent on one another, such that psychological illnesses have physical manifestations and vice versa. Although similar views have historically been important in Western traditions, their place does not extend to modern times, unlike in Iran, where such historical conceptualisations remain influential to the present day. In discussions of melancholia, first articulated by Al-Razi and expanded on by Ibn-Sina (or Avicenna), this interdependency is seen clearly. For instance, Ibn-Sina attributes one of the causes of melancholia to the domination of one of the humours on the brain, thus causing an imbalance that results in sadness, overthinking, anger, and isolation. With this characterisation, the best way to try to cure such an imbalance would be through a change in diet to restore the balance of the humours (Avicenna 1999/1025). However, he argues that melancholic characteristics are not exclusively rooted in humoral imbalances in the brain, but can originate in various parts of the body, as well as being caused by psychological factors such as excessive fear and grief. Different causes of the imbalance, in this view, merit different treatments (Al-Issa 2000, p. 48). Ibn-Sina tried to explain the physiological mechanisms that give rise to melancholic characteristics. For example, he claims these could be due to "the whole body's black-bile intemperament or the dysfunction of the major organs, particularly the spleen, liver, and the stomach, for various reasons … Ibn-Sīnā emphasises the heart; its cold and dry intemperament was, according to him, a frequent cause of melancholia – at least it was impossible for the heart not to be associated in some way when such a temperament affected another part of the body" (Dols 1992, p. 81). These accounts make clear the emphasis placed on the body in investigating psychological ailments, and in particular the importance attached to the heart.

The historical trajectory between melancholia and depression has been noted in various studies (e.g. Radden 2003, 2009) and is not exclusive to Iranian/Islamic medicine. However, what is noteworthy is the present-day place of traditional medicine in Iran and the continuing influence of conceptions explored in this tradition on the folk theories around health and illness which continue to play a part in everyday thinking and behaviours of Iranians in encounters with illness. In other words, traditional medicine, its characterisation of illness, and the remedies it offers for various ailments, form part of the Iranian culture. This is true to such an extent that Iranians continue to refer to traditional texts for everyday ailments and their cure, and everyone has at least a basic grasp of the claims and arguments made by traditional medicine. The continuing influence of this field is further evidenced by the creation of new institutions dedicated to teaching and researching Iranian and Islamic medicine. It is due to this familiarity that, when it comes to mental illness, Iranians tend to accept claims that are in line with their belief system; for example that exercising, as a form of taking care of one's physical health, is effective in ensuring one's mental health, given the interdependency of the two. On the other hand, various claims and practices which are further away from the engrained belief system are met with stronger resistance, such as the idea that there might be an illness characterised purely by psychological distress, or that antidepressants might be an effective treatment of depression. It should be noted that the use of chemical medicine for physical illness is an accepted form of medicine in Iran, despite its divergence from traditional medicine, due to the long history of its practice in the country as well as familiarity with its effectiveness. The same cannot be said for medicine used for mental illness, and there remains a degree of scepticism regarding such treatments, as seen in the earlier discussions in Chap. 5.

Given the place of traditional medicine, not only in practice, but in ways of thinking and interpreting illness in Iran, ideas about depression are highly influenced by these pre-existing systems of belief. Stigmatisation of depression in Iranian society arises from the inability to accept a mental illness which is not accompanied by physical symptoms. This leads a large portion of patients with depression to feel the burden of having to legitimise their illness, and many come to report physical symptoms, as discussed in the case of uncontrollable crying. Such way of thinking partly explains why the emphasis on somatic symptoms is higher in Iran as compared to the UK. This view is confirmed by a practicing psychiatrist in Iran who told me that although Iranians have no problem talking about their emotional and psychological suffering, they often feel that their suffering can only be acknowledged if accompanied by somatic symptoms. This emphasis, furthermore, is seen more among patients from less affluent backgrounds, such as small villages, where there is higher stigma attached to mental illnesses such as depression. In larger cities, however, such as Shiraz and Tehran, complaints of somatic symptoms are seen less frequently, or do not carry the same heavy emphasis (Moghimi 2017—personal correspondence).

What is evident is the role of folk theories of illness, which not only account for the roots of the stigmatisation of depression in Iran, but also offer a way of explaining the presence of somatic symptoms in patients. In other words, those suffering from depression, by virtue of understanding the dominant frames of thought, consciously or otherwise, know that by the cultural conceptions of illness dominant in society, an illness such as depression is legitimised and made more understandable if accompanied by somatic symptoms. The cultural frames of thought in this regard act as a space of shared understanding in which individuals can seek one another's acceptance by adhering to shared values and systems of beliefs. Although such mechanisms are not necessarily carried out consciously, they remain part of the way in which individuals conduct themselves and adhere to the accepted norms and values of the collective society.

Such stigma-avoiding communication strategies are not unique to Iran. As the body of literature on somatisation of depression among Chinese patients shows, knowledge of the expectations of society and ways of escaping stigmatisation plausibly plays an important role in the higher levels of reported somatic symptoms in China. In this case, knowledge of how different symptoms are interpreted in society, leads to communication strategies designed to avoid certain outcomes, such as stigmatisation. It is also important to note that in accounting for Chinese somatisation, studies point either to variation in the actual experience and expression of distress, or to variation in the understanding of particular symptoms and their significance and the communication of this understanding to others (Ryder and Chentsova-Dutton 2012). This distinction, however, overlooks the fact that social and learned understandings of illness and/

or various symptoms influence the individual's lived experience of the symptoms.

> In any given cultural context, a specific symptom might attract social support, bring shame on the family, provide rapid access to health care resources, be politically threatening, or indeed have any number of different consequences. These realities do not simply provide sufferers with a menu of behavioral options, but rather shape which aspects of the phenomenal field are attended to and then emphasized. Different social worlds draw out different symptoms. (Zhou et al. 2016, p. 5)

These two seemingly distinct elements, therefore, are equally important in understanding and accounting for somatisation in cross-cultural studies.

In the Iranian understanding, psychological and physical symptoms of an illness, rather than being separate and distinct, are together constitutive of the overall experience of illness. Such a conceptualisation comes in contrast to the dominant Western views which see the body and bodily feelings as fundamentally distinct from the mental and psychological, with the central presumption that the body only serves as a vessel for projecting the inner states of the mind and the psyche. As Fuchs has noted, in this Western conceptualisation, somatisation "denotes a shift of psychological content or meaning onto the body, leading to the rather Eurocentric view that members of non-Western cultures have only insufficient introspective or verbal capacities to perceive and express their feelings in a mature way" (Fuchs 2014, p. 184). In a culture such as Iran, however, rather than being an extra culturally specific symptom of depression, somatic symptoms ought to be viewed as an essential integral part of the experience of depression. Although the misconceptions and the resultant stigmatisation of depression demands the existence of somatic symptoms in depression, the starting point of both the stigmatisation and the significance of somatic symptoms for the individual experiencing them, remain the same; namely, the cultural conceptualisation of illness, which views physical and psychological symptoms as essentially integral parts of the whole experience of the illness. This unity of psychological and physical symptoms means that the significance of somatic symptoms, as well as being a way of avoiding stigmas, lies in the lived experience of patients. Viewed as an essential part of the experience of depression, somatic symptoms therefore ought to be analysed in terms of the phenomenology of embodiment and the significance of the body as the primary point of contact between the individual and the world in which she dwells.

Somatic Symptoms as Disturbances to Embodiment

The body, or a certain part of it, is central in the experience of different states that are referred to as 'feelings', ranging from feelings of touch to existential feelings, which form the basis of our relation to the world. As the medium through which we find ourselves and our being-in-the-world, the body constitutes a central aspect of our experience in the world. Notably, not only is the body the medium through which we perceive and experience the world, but is itself an object of perception that resides in the world. This twofold characteristic of the body was noted most distinctly by Merleau-Ponty:

> If it is true that I am conscious of my body through the world and if my body is the unperceived term at the center of the world toward which every object turns its face, then it is true for the same reason that my body is the pivot of the world … it is as though our body comprises two distinct layers, that of the habitual body and that of the actual body. (Merleau-Ponty 2012/1945, p. 84)

This important phenomenological distinction, in other words, is "between the body that I prereflectively live, that is, the lived or subject body (Leib), and the physical body that I can perceive or that is perceived by others, in other words, the object body (Körper)" (Fuchs and Schlimme 2009, pp. 570–571). This distinction can also be seen in the way we relate to the world through our bodily feelings. As Ratcliffe shows, whilst "some feelings reveal parts of the body in an object-like way, … others operate as a medium through which something else is experienced"

(Ratcliffe 2008, p. 107). In experiencing some feelings we experience the body as an object of perception or experience, whilst in others, the body itself is the subject *doing* the perceiving or experiencing of an object residing out there in the world.

As such, not only is the body the primary source of our self-experience, but it also serves as the medium of our contact with the world. Therefore, background bodily feelings such as tension or relaxation, ease or unease, affect the way in which the world is presented to us, by colouring all world-directed experiences (Fuchs 2014), by virtue of the body being the means through which we perceive and experience the world. Understood in this way, not only is the lived body directed outwards towards things in the world, but it also "opens up the world as a space of purposive, practical possibilities, and thus shapes all our experiences, activities and thoughts" (Ratcliffe 2008, p. 107). The centrality of the body and bodily experiences motivate an account of depression in terms of bodily experiences which are disrupted in the course of the illness. Disruptions in our embodied experiences of ourselves and the world we live in, on such an account, encompasses not only the physical sensations involved in depression, but also our affective experiences and relations with others.

Disturbances of embodiment, following the phenomenological distinction between object body and subject body, can be classified into two main forms. In the first instance, disturbance of embodiment can be related to explicit body awareness or one's body image and can therefore be seen as disturbance related to object body. Disturbances understood in this sense, seen for example in cases of anorexia nervosa, signify conscious perceptions, emotions and attitudes towards one's body. On the second classification, disturbances of embodiment affect the subject body, i.e. the pre-reflective embodied sense of self. This latter form of disturbance can be seen in schizophrenia and depression, where one's sense of self is diminished, or one's contact with the world, as primarily a bodily experience, is altered.

#27(F) – I feel like my body gets heavy.
#7(F) – [I feel] numb/leaden. Without energy. Sleepy. Endless hunger.
#4(F) – [I feel] beaten (*koofteh*), tired, bent (*khamideh*).

#35(F) – My physical ability decreases, but because of the conditions of my life I have to carry on working.
#33(M) – [I feel] lethargy, listlessness, feeling weak [to do] daily social tasks.
#42(M) – I feel that my body is weak and numb.
#25(M) – I don't have any feelings [in my body].

One of the most common embodied experiences of depression, seen equally in Iran and the UK, which can illuminate on the nature of the disturbance of embodiment affecting the subject body, is the perception of the body as heavy and leaden, or weak and numb (see Ratcliffe 2015, p. 76). The body in this sense loses its quality of fluidity and transparency as a medium of experience and becomes instead a solid, leaden body which, instead of giving access to the world and one's surroundings, presents an obstacle to the individual's desires, intentions and impulses, such that "phenomenal space is not embodied anymore" (Fuchs and Schlimme 2009, p. 572). In experiencing the overwhelming sense of fatigue and physical weakness, as felt in depression, the patient is confronted with her body, not as a medium of which she is only prereflectively aware, but as a limiting and oppressive force. The limiting quality of the body in depression influences the way in which one relates to the world, such that its confining nature reflects the loss of possibilities and the limiting nature of the world as felt by depressed patients. "The open horizon of possible experiences shrinks into a locked atmosphere, in which everything becomes permeated by a sense of lost possibilities" (Fuchs and Schlimme 2009, pp. 572–573).

The perception of the body as heavy and leaden, numb and weak, can be thought of as a form of disturbance of embodiment seen universally across cultures to an extent that "one may conclude that depression is primarily experienced as a *bodily disturbance* in a majority of cultures, rather than only shifted and projected to the body secondarily" (Fuchs 2014, p. 183). However, the physical sensations in depression are varied and different feelings are complained about to different degrees in different cultures. One example of such a variation is in the presence of pain in various parts of the body. Ratcliffe reports some complaints made by patients in the UK, of general aches and pains, joint pain, and headaches

(Ratcliffe 2015, p. 75). Although such complaints form a small percentage of the complaints regarding physical symptoms in the UK sample, similar complaints in the Iranian sample are seen much more frequently. In fact, in the Iranian sample, complaints of pain are the most frequent complaints of physical discomfort, after complaints of fatigue and physical weakness. This difference can be accounted for not only through the social pressures and stigmas that demand an easily understandable physical symptom such as pain, but also through the culturally specific attitudes and behaviours towards the sensation of pain itself. Yet pain is primarily felt and experienced on an individual domain, and only secondarily put in the cultural domain of understanding and interpretation through its expression and communication. As such, a phenomenological account of pain experience should be laid out before turning to culture, as a meaning-making system for interpretation of these individual experiences, and as the background that gives these experiences their significance.

#17(F) – I sleep a lot, I have headaches, my body feels heavy.
#14(F) – [I have] feelings of excessive exhaustion and headaches, together with lack of appetite and physical weakness.
#36 – I feel shattered, and I often have body pain and am completely frustrated (*asabi*).
#29(F) – [I have] neck pain, hand trembling.
#8 (M)– I have disc herniation … constant back ache and [feeling] shattered. When I'm in a good mood I work three times more than a normal person.
#20(F) – I have pain in my arms and legs, I sleep a lot more.
#19(F) – Feeling of feebleness (*hes-e bi-hāli*), headaches and crying.

The experience of bodily pains in depression is documented in different cultures (e.g. Drehera et al. 2017; Bair and Robinson 2003). The International Association for the Study of Pain defines it as "An unpleasant sensory and emotional experience associated with actual or potential tissue damage, or described in terms of such damage" (IASP 2017), making clear the inseparability of the bodily sensation of pain from the emotional experience of being in pain. As an emotional experience, expressions and understanding of pain are learned and occur and find meaning within a social, cultural, and linguistic context. Indeed, empirical cross-cultural studies support this claim, noting that "Culture is the conditioning influence in forming the individual's patterns of responding to and expressing pain" (Lovering 2006, p. 390). The various studies on cultures and histories of pain attest to the multifaceted nature of the experience, as well as the complexity of its relationship in any given cultural or historical context (e.g. Bending 2000; Moscoso 2012; Bourke 2014).

In his discussion of the phenomenology of chronic pain, Fredrik Svenaeus puts forward a phenomenological account of pain as an embodied experience encompassing both emotional and physical domains of experience (Svenaeus 2015). Emphasising the experiential aspect of pain—that pain is primarily suffered rather than known, Svenaeus highlights the nature of the experience of pain as an awareness of one's body in illness. As noted in the discussion of unhomelikeness, in illness one's relationship with the world is altered, and this includes one's perception of, and relation to one's own body. In illness one is more aware of the limiting qualities of one's body and the effort with which previously undemanding tasks are carried out. Svenaeus construes the experience of pain as an example of the way in which the body, and more specifically suffering in the body, is brought to the centre of one's consciousness. The suffering brought about in pain, Svenaeus argues, can be described "as a kind of *bodily resistance and modulation* displaying itself at the heart of consciousness and human experience" (Svenaeus 2015, p. 113). Just in the case of various bodily sensations in illness, one is confronted here with a sense of alienation from one's own body, since the suffering in pain presents "an awareness of a body that is mine, but yet alien, since it resists and disturbs, rather than supports, my ways of being conscious and directed towards the world" (ibid.). Construed in this way, one can begin to see parallels with accounts of disturbance of embodiment in depression. Just as in the case of the perception of the body as heavy and leaden, which rather than disclosing, *encloses* the world in which one dwells, the individual in pain experiences her body as alien, one that upsets the normal harmony between desires, intentions, and possibilities for action.

The experience of being-in-pain has an all-encompassing nature; as a world-enclosing sensation, pain directs the individual's focus towards her body, as a body in pain, which would otherwise remain in the background of experiences. Svenaeus describes this shift in consciousness by construing pain as a mood which permeates our entire being-in-the-world. In experiencing the mood of pain, he argues, "the world literally disappears; our horizon of meaningfulness gradually shrinks until nothing but the self-centred pain remains" (Svenaeus 2015, p. 116)). Of course, this description, being concerned with chronic pain experiences, strikes one as too strong a claim to be applied to pain as an instance of somatised depression. However, the fact remains that in experiencing any kind of pain, the sensation becomes the centre of one's attention and in so doing influences a range of thoughts and activities that determine one's relationship to the world. The inability to carry out the daily tasks and what is routinely expected of one, as felt in depression, can in large part be attributed to the disturbance of embodiment. This is since a large part of other symptoms seen in depression, such as lack of motivation and drive towards the daily activities, manifest themselves in bodily sensations as well, as has been seen in the case of heavy and leaden body in depression. Therefore, pain in various parts of the body, feelings of weakness and fatigue, and the perception of the body as heavy and leaden, can all be thought of as various instances in which the body and awareness of it comes to the foreground of one's consciousness as a limiting factor in everything one does. In all these instances the body, previously the enabling medium for experiences and navigating the world, presents an impenetrable obstacle to one's normal way of being and relating to the world.

Such phenomenological significance of the sensation of pain, which colours the way the individual in pain relates to the world and to her body as the medium for experiences, precedes the sociocultural understanding and significance of pain. But the observation that our individual experiences are always situated within a given sociocultural context, one that dominates our framework for understanding and interpretation, means that individuals understand their individual experiences of pain against this broader cultural context. If presence of pain is seen more or less universally across different cultures, what makes this symptom significant in a given cultural context? What makes pain one of the most complained about symptom of depression in Iran, when it is only mentioned in passing in the UK?

In the first instance, in accounting for the experience of pain among the Iranian sample, pain should be understood as a potentially expressive sensation. The sociocultural beliefs and attitudes towards pain, which vary cross culturally, give meaning to the experience of pain. As Kleinman argues, somatisation can be thought of as a "habitual *coping style* or *idiom of distress*" (Kleinman and Kleinman 1985, p. 473), learned through one's experience of living in a certain sociocultural setting. The multifaceted nature of pain experience is also captured in the 'social communication model' of pain, which in addition to the biological and/or psychological nature of pain, recognises pain *experience* as facilitated through inter- and intrapersonal factors, thus acknowledging the complexities of the phenomenon of pain, including:

> the very complex biology of tissue injury and repair; the complexities of the experience of pain; the varyingly public verbal, nonverbal, and physiological manifestations of pain; the complex reactions of observers as they endeavour to appraise and understand the person's pain; and the complex judgements associated with decisions to deliver or withhold care, amongst other possibilities. (Craig 2009, p. 23)

Understanding pain as an instance of somatisation, therefore, requires an understanding of social attitudes and understanding of pain within a given culture, in addition to the embodied experience of pain. As seen from Svenaeus' account, pain is characterised by the debilitating effect it has on an individual's normal way of being-in-the-world. This effect plays a significant role in explaining the common understandings of, and behaviours towards experiences of pain in Iranian culture. Within this context, pain is regarded as a highly debilitating phenomenon with an all-encompassing character which takes over one's normal way of being. An individual in pain, therefore, is not faced with the same expectations and is rather viewed more sympathetically and compassionately by others. Due to this understanding of pain, it is common for individuals to use being in pain as an excuse and/or an explanation for one's inability to perform certain actions or be a certain way. For instance, a simple headache can be an acceptable reason for one's unwillingness or inability to engage in social gatherings or doing a task expected of them. What adds to this understanding, is arguably the familiarity of the sensation of pain, which readily arouses feelings of sympathy in others, and in so doing, allows the individual in pain to use her pain experience as an explanatory tool for her behaviour and state of being. In this context then, being in pain, or the expression of being such, can be thought of as a means of standing out from others and getting noticed, which would mean that the usual rules and expectations no longer apply to one.

Such an understanding of pain is also partly explained by some of the cultural norms and attitudes towards pain relief in Iran. Although there are very few studies conducted on pain culture in Iran, scattered medical investigations provide some insight into the matter. A survey of cancer patients, for instance, demonstrates a desire to tolerate pain, and the belief that unless the pain is unbearable, one should refrain from taking pain killers (Najafi Ghezeljeh and Hosseini 2012). Of those surveyed, 69% agreed with the statement that 'before asking for a painkiller one should wait for the pain to become really severe', while 63% agreed that 'painkillers should only be used when pain is at its severest'. Such attitudes can be broken down to three elements, namely, attitudes towards painkillers, beliefs regarding the ability to control pain severity through mental strength, and the cultural beliefs that suffering pain can be good for one.

Painkillers are readily available for purchase in Iran, including strong and potentially addictive ones that may require a prescription in other countries. The study mentioned above reveals the prevalence of inaccurate beliefs about such medications that in part explains the patients' reluctance towards taking them. For instance, a large percentage of patients believe that painkillers *generally* are extremely addictive (77.5%), with a larger percentage believing that there is a possibility of getting addicted to painkillers (79%). Additionally, over half of those studied (59.5%) believe that using painkillers for minor pain means that these would not be effective in reducing severe pains later on. What is considered to be an effective way of alleviating pain among this sample is individual mental strength and wellbeing. A large majority of the patients under study believe that thinking about pain increases the severity of pain

(80.5%), and that the severity of pain can be controlled by changing one's thoughts (72.5%). Similarly, 88% believe that depressed feeling and mood worsens pain, and conversely, 89% believe that tolerating pain is much easier in a state of calmness and equanimity.

Lastly, and perhaps most importantly, are the prevalent cultural beliefs regarding the relationship between tolerating pain and having a strong (and sometimes righteous) character, which makes one stand out from others. In line with the beliefs discussed earlier, that suffering is an inevitable part of life and one's attempts to be a good person, suffering from pain can be understood as a means to strengthening one's character and act as an atonement for one's sins. Such beliefs can be invoked in accounting for some of the beliefs regarding the nature and use of painkillers as well. If one is in pain and believes that tolerating this pain makes her stand out from others and can be seen as having a strong character, not only is there incentive for her not to take painkillers, but also to express her being in pain more openly. Within a community that shares such an understanding, an individual in pain would also be received by others with more sympathy and compassion. In a context where social misunderstandings and misjudgements about depression determine a depressed individuals' mood and experiences, an emphasis on feelings of pain can be a means of receiving more sympathy and understanding from others.

These prevalent beliefs and attitudes towards pain and reactions to it reveal the expressiveness of pain experience and the notion of agency and personal worth attached to it. Part of the significance of the higher emphasis on pain among Iranian depressed patients can be explained once it is established that, for cultural reasons people are more reluctant to take painkillers, and instead more open to express and talk about their experience of being in pain—in order to arouse empathy or understanding in others, for instance. Prohibitive attitudes towards painkillers, such as their being addictive or losing effectiveness with time, can be thought to legitimate higher emphasis and expression of pain experience, leading to one's character and status standing out among others, and higher levels of empathy in others.

Indeed, as noted earlier, Iranians often make use of physical sensations to express emotional distress and the physical sensation of pain can indeed be seen as an example of this sort of expression. In a qualitative study of chronic lower back pain among Iranian women, for instance, we see not only that the women attribute the cause of their pain to emotional distress resulting from difficulties of life and the pressure they find themselves under, but also that the pain itself gave voice to these difficulties and was expressed as an idiom of distress (Tavafian et al. 2008, p. 343). Additionally, the participants in the study linked their back pain with their emotions: "back pain became a proxy indicator of emotional upset. It was akin to an 'emotions barometer'" (ibid.).

Now it is given these observations, regarding the significance of the experience of pain both on an individual as well as socio-cultural levels, that the significance of the sensation of pain as presented in depression can be understood. As pointed out earlier, the stigmatisation of depression as a mental illness and the social expectations of such an illness play an important role in somatisation of depression in Iran. The stigmas are often based around the understanding of illness, as construed in traditional medicine, which emphasises the interdependency of physical and mental or emotional symptoms. As seen in Chap. 5, Iranian depressed patients often complain of the fact that others find it difficult to accept an illness such as depression which does not manifest with physical, observable symptoms. Given the understanding of pain in Iranian culture, the presence of pain in the experience of depression enables patients to escape at least some of the stigmatisation. In other words, not only does the sensation of pain—much in the same way as uncontrollable crying discussed in Chap. 5—act as a legitimising factor for depression as a 'real' illness, but it also removes the expectations of others that the patient in depression is unable to meet. The presence of the sensation of pain, given its nature as taking over all aspects of one's life and relation to the world, acts as an explanatory tool for why the patient in depression is unable to do the daily tasks or be her usual self, in a way that removes the blame from the individual and acknowledges the nature of depression as an illness that affects all aspects of one's being.

It is important to note that the explanatory power of the sensation of pain, and the legitimising effect it has for depression as a 'real' illness, does not undermine the phenomenological significance of the sensation for the patient herself. On the contrary, the two aspects of the experience can be thought of as interdependent and complementary. It is because pain is experienced as an all-encompassing sensation, one that disturbs one's usual understanding of the body and its abilities, that the patient is able to link the sensation to her altered abilities and behaviours. On the other hand, the communication of the state of one in pain and the link between pain and the disruption it causes is made possible given the background of shared sociocultural understanding of pain as a debilitating experience that influences all aspects of one's life.

Cross-cultural variation in presentation with and complaints of somatic symptoms in depression once again demonstrate the importance of seeing phenomenological and cultural elements alongside one another. While phenomenological considerations allow us to view somatic symptoms as part of the embodied experience of depression, the significance attached to the experience of these symptoms, including how they are interpreted and communicated, is tied to cultural conceptions and social expectations. Whether we are concerned with the universal disturbance to embodiment in depression, or cultural variation in specific somatic symptoms such as presentation with pain, it is essential that the experience is situated within a culturally significant context. It is the totality of these cultural factors that determine the significance of somatic symptoms in depression. Therefore, accounts which attempt to reduce the complex and interdependent nature of these elements into a simple difference between Western and non-Western cultures, or the ability or inability to express emotional and psychological distress, fail to capture the important place of somatic symptoms in depression in its entirety.

8

Culture, Experiences and Narratives, and the Problem of Interpretation

The preceding analysis has been an attempt at providing a plausible account of how depressive experiences are created in the image of cultural modes of understanding. Cultural scripts and understandings, as meaning-making systems, are fluid and ever-evolving, thus giving rise to myriad ways of shaping and reshaping experiences and individuals' understanding of them. It is nevertheless undeniable that cultural conceptions and ways of thought and interpretation have a considerable influence on the way a phenomenon such as depression is experienced. Embedded within this claim, and indeed within the methodological approach of the work, is the inseparability of narratives of experience, themselves culturally shaped, from the experiences themselves. This inseparability is manifested in most of the symptoms examined in this work, albeit to different extents. In the analyses presented, the starting point has been the first-person accounts, i.e. the way individuals themselves talk about their experiences. From these personal narratives, cultural models of thought, and frameworks for interpretation are extracted, and it is these cultural elements that are shown to be largely underlying the variation in the experiences of depression. This qualitative account, however, begs the question as to how this interdependency ought to be

M. Mirdamadi, *A Phenomenological Study of Depression in Iran*,
https://doi.org/10.1007/978-3-031-30407-1_8

understood on a theoretical level, with the potential to be applied to future cross-cultural studies.

I suggest that we ought to understand experiences as fundamentally bound with culture, and cultural narratives. In this penultimate chapter a theoretical sketch for such an understanding is offered, one which can be shown to be compatible not only with anthropological accounts of the link between experiences and culture, but also with the phenomenological views of experiences and the nature of our relation to the world. As I demonstrate, however, certain notions are rendered obsolete within such a conceptualisation—notably that of idioms of distress, which loses its explanatory power as a tool for understanding culturally unique behaviours.

Culture, Narratives, and Experience

The close connection and interplay between narratives, experiences and culture can be demonstrated by means of an example. Consider cross-cultural variation in experiences of grief—that is, the way in which different groups of people, *by virtue of their culture,* talk about and experience the same phenomenon in different ways. The conceptualisation of death in Iran, as well as the rituals following someone's death, are based on a religious framework, where death is viewed as a passing from one world to the next. The funeral ceremony, therefore, is organised so as to respect and address the religious beliefs. Furthermore, in a collectivist society like Iran, where the death of someone close is a significant event, the ceremonies present a space for those who remain to mourn in a way that suits the norms and customs of the group. The rituals start with family members burying the dead, not in a coffin, but wrapped in a white cloth (*kafan*), which could become loose, revealing to the grieving crowd the dead person's face or arm as they are burying them. The custom demands that the mourning rituals take place on an ongoing basis for a year, with those close to the lost one refusing to take off their black clothes for the period. The rituals, filled with grieving chants and songs, and with women crying and screaming, take place on the day of the burial, as well as on the third, seventh, and fortieth day since the burial, and are concluded with a gathering on the anniversary of the burial. Needless to say, the normal course of life is interrupted, not only because of the immense sense of sadness one feels after a loss, but also due to the cultural norms, which necessitate the planning and preparing the ceremonies and accommodating for the often-large number of people attending.

Now in comparing the experiences of loss by two sets of individuals, one from Iran and other from the UK, it has to be acknowledged that their experiences are not limited to an internal feeling with no influence from the outside world. Cultural ways of understanding and interpreting the phenomena of loss and death, shape the way people experience the phenomenon, as well as their expressions and interpretation of the experiences, both in the moment and in later recollections. Embedded within any personal account of experiences, are the cultural conceptions and customs which shape the individual experiences of loss, regardless of whether associations and links are made explicitly and consciously or not. It is in this sense that the way loss is experienced in a given culture is inherently and essentially cultural. Consequently, any attempt at understanding these experiences and their variation across cultures needs to take into account the cultural setting that shapes experiences and narratives, in order to get a comprehensive picture of various factors influencing the overall experiences. Furthermore, in the absence of phenomenological access to the different ways of experiencing, there is nothing else that can be known and/or studied about the way an individual or a collective experience a phenomenon, except for the cultural background of experiences which account for the understanding and interpretation of the phenomenon experienced.

Experiences and narratives, rather than separate and operating on different levels of primacy, ought to be viewed as closely and deeply intertwined: "for experience structures expressions, in that we understand other people and their expressions on the basis of our own experience and self-understanding. But expressions also structure experience, in that dominant narratives of a historical era, important rituals and festivals, and classic works of art [thus the cultural context] define and illuminate inner experience" (Bruner 1986, p. 6). This relational link between narratives and experiences is not due to one being a copy of the other, but because of what Mattingly (1998) calls a 'structural homology' between the two. The close link between narratives and experiences can be illustrated through understanding the role of culture as a mediator between experiences and narratives. The 'structural homology' Mattingly refers to, can be seen to be a result of this role of culture, as influencing both and providing a context in terms of which experiences are understood and narratives are created.

This defining role of culture is accounted for most clearly in the works of Clifford Geertz, through the emphasis placed on cultural structures as having a meaning-making role for both experiences and narratives. What is important for our discussion is Geertz's characterisation of cultural processes, not as something that happens 'in the head', but rather as structures of significance that "impose meaning upon experience" (Geertz 1973, p. 45). These are not 'in the head' in the sense that they transcend the individuals' frames of thought and are constitutive of the world where individuals dwell, therefore shaping the background against which they understand and interpret their experiences. In this sense culture is construed as an organising force that shapes our experiences and gives meaning and significance to them, such that without culture "man's behaviour would be virtually ungovernable, a mere chaos of pointless acts and exploding emotions, his experience virtually shapeless" (ibid., p. 46). This role of culture as conditioning for experiences means that it is fundamentally impossible to separate experiences from the cultural settings that give rise to them. Similarly, by providing the context for understanding experiences, culture shapes the narratives of experience, as a tool through which the understanding of an experience is made possible.

There is additionally a temporal element to the cultural domain of experience. This is since the norms and practices that shape the culture, and the norms and modes of understanding which link the cultural context to the experiences of a phenomenon, come about in a historical context (e.g. Hacking 2002). This temporal element has been an important point in the approach of the present study, since in many instances the strong cultural elements that influence experiences of depression can be traced historically. Indeed, some of the strongest cultural elements in this domain are those with a long history which has allowed them to shape part of the conceptual framework of the society in its encounter with depression—as is the case with traditional medicine and the folk beliefs arising from it.

One theoretical notion that aims to bring together history, cultural practices and experiences of a phenomenon is Pierre Bourdieu's *habitus.*[1] For Bourdieu, this notion provides a means for reconciling the social structure of the world with individual agency, and aims to account for the way the 'outer' social life and the 'inner' self, shape and reshape one another (Maton 2008).[2] In addition to placing emphasis on the role of the cultural and social context in the construction of individual conceptions and practices, habitus explains the way these practices change through time and thus provides a link between the past, present and future practices.

The habitus is understood primarily as a property of social agents, and in terms of the individual's dispositions, which Bourdieu defines as a kind of structure; a way of being or a habitual state that incorporates individual inclinations and tendencies (Bourdieu 1977, p. 214). As the internalisation of social structures and norms, dispositions are the carriers of history into the present and future practices. The habitus is therefore defined as a "system of durable, transposable dispositions" (Bourdieu 1990, p. 53), with the power of generating and maintaining practices. As a property of social agents, moreover, habitus comprises a "structured, and structuring, structure" (Bourdieu 1994, p. 170). It is structured in the sense that it is comprised of one's past and present circumstances, and structuring since it shapes, or at least helps in the shaping of, one's present and future practices. And lastly, it is a structure itself in that it is regulated and systematically ordered, as opposed to being random and disorganised (Maton 2008, p. 51). The habitus thus incorporates the element of temporality in sociocultural ways of being, thinking, and acting.

[1] Ian Hacking has also suggested an account of understanding phenomena and our experience of them in a historical context (Hacking 2002), and has shown how the historical developments change our perceptions and understanding of some mental disorders (Hacking 1995). I use Bourdieu's account in detailing this link, as his account is concerned with history, as well as cultural norms and customs. Thus the links between his account and the arguments presented in this work can be drawn more easily.

[2] Note the parallels between this theory and the importance of outer and inner self in the Iranian culture and its influence on the conceptions and experiences of interpersonal relationships, as noted in Chap. 2.

The habitus further generates individuals' perceptions, beliefs, and appreciation of the *field*, i.e. the social and cultural context that individuals inhabit. It is important to note here, the importance of the field in the process of generating practices and beliefs: it is the relational nature, and the interdependency of field and habitus that gives rise to these practices. The field, Bourdieu claims, presents itself to the individuals as a 'space of possibles' defined with respect to the individual's position in the field. These possibilities then become operative and active as achievable possibilities, "in so far as they are perceived and appreciated through the schemes of perception and appreciation which constitute a habitus" (Bourdieu 1993, p. 64). In other words, the habitus, as a cognitive system for perception, appreciation, and formation of practices and beliefs is constructed in accordance with the field one inhabits, and one's position within it, while the space of possibilities embedded in the field are actualised in accordance with one's habitus, thus indicating the interdependent relation of the two. In talking about the variation in rituals of burial and the experience of grief in Iran, one can see that the centrality of religion, and the place of interpersonal relationships in the Iranian culture, as well as the emphasis on the public display of sadness in the society, define the space for the formation of the specific rituals of burial and mourning. In other words, it is against the backdrop of sociocultural values and belief systems that particular practices find meaning and significance.

As such, the habitus explains not only the individual's practices and beliefs, but also the collective, regulated practices and conceptions found in groups of people. As a system encompassing "principles of the generation and structuring of practices and representations" (Bourdieu 1977, p. 72), the habitus gives rise to regulated practices, without this regulation being the result of obedience to rules that exist objectively in the society. Rather, these are "collectively orchestrated without being the product of the orchestrating action of a conductor" (ibid.). The regulated and orchestrated nature of practices is due to them being the product of collective past experiences and conditions of being, which produce the principles underlying the present practices. The harmonising effect of the habitus is seen more clearly among groups of people that share a similar position in the field, and are therefore likely to have similar experiences, leading to similar beliefs and perceptions.

Consider the example of generational memories of the Iran-Iraq war. For those growing up in the war, although elements of the experiences would be different (e.g. proximity to war zones), they share a largely similar position in the field. As such, as Behrouzan (2016) has shown, many of the conceptions, beliefs, and perceptions held by those with similar experiences of the war, or similar memories of these experiences, are comparable in form, and influential in shaping present principles, sense of identity and experiences of phenomena. Bourdieu argues that this similarity in experiences as a result of a common structure, leads to the harmony seen in the collective practices and conceptions, since similar experiences give rise to similar principles in the habitus, which in turn shape future practices among the group. These similarities, furthermore, define for these members a common sense of reality and a common anticipated future. As such, practices produced by the habitus can be accounted for through the relation between these practices and social conditions, which gave rise to the principles producing these practices, thus relating the past to the present. It is in this sense that for Bourdieu, habitus is "history turned into nature" (Bourdieu 1977, p. 78).

The creation of a common-sense world is an important effect of the orchestration of habitus. In such a world, through consensus within the group, practices and conceptions are deemed sensible and reasonable. This consensus comes from "the harmonization of agents' experiences and the continuous reinforcement that each of them receives from the expression, individual or collective, improvised or programmed, of similar or identical experiences" (Bourdieu 1977, p. 80). Construed as such, the habitus not only incorporates the history and the past experiences and conceptions into the present ones, but also defines a framework through which commonalities in beliefs and practices among members of a society and culture, and their significance, can be understood and accounted for.

To summarise, Bourdieu's analysis starts with an account of dispositions as a way of being, incorporating individuals' tendencies and inclinations, with regards to both perceptions and interpretations of experiences, and the resulting actions and practices. These dispositions, being the product of past experiences and beliefs, lay the foundations for the formation of principles and cognitive schemas, i.e. the habitus, which has the power of generating new practices, beliefs, perceptions and interpretations. As a consequence of being the product of dispositions, as the internalisations of the structures of the society and past experiences, the collective habitus is harmonised and orchestrated. This is such that members of the same social group are endowed with a system of meaning, that renders the world they inhabit and their practices meaningful and sensible. In this way, then, the habitus is a product of history. However, it also has the power of shaping the future, since it is in accordance with the habitus and the practice-generating principles within it, that certain possibilities presented to the individuals within the field are activated with the potential to be actualised.

Culture, therefore, as a system of practices, beliefs, and a way of being in and relating to the world, is seen to be intimately linked with individual and collective history and memories, giving the world a sense of meaning. In accounting for the way depression is conceptualised and encountered in a culture, it is important to note the various factors, not only those that in the present are seen to influence narratives and experiences of depression, but also those with historical significance, which give the present narratives and encounters their meaning. The way depression is understood, experienced, and articulated in Iran today, is a result of cultural ways of understanding (e.g. death-consciousness), which are themselves shaped and influenced by shared historical events (e.g. Iran-Iraq war). Taking note of temporality in the discussion is also important in accounting for change in encounters with depression. As societies change and go through different shared experiences, so do the beliefs and perceptions of phenomena and events and could result in major cultural shifts. The findings and analyses in the present work is considerably different to those conducted in Iran before the 1979 revolution, in part due to such cultural shifts.

In conducting a phenomenological study, although the prime focus of study is experiences, it must be acknowledged that these experiences are had by an individual as a being-in-the-world. When we talk about 'the world of depression' and the 'existential change' involved in depression, we aim to signify a change in the way an individual in depression understands herself and the world around her. Yet it is important to note that this change in perception does not happen in isolation but is rather dependent on how the individual understands herself and her place in the world, as well as the way she understands depression itself. Various factors, such as culture, history, language, and politics, shape the background of understanding and way of thought for individuals. A phenomenological understanding of depression is therefore incomplete without considering these meaning-making factors, especially in a cross-cultural study aiming to understand variations in experiences.

There are various methodological consequences of this understanding. First and foremost, as I have already demonstrated, it is important to recognise individuals and the way they understand and articulate their experiences as *situated* within a phenomenologically significant context. This context is constituted by cultural ways of thought and understanding, shaped by historical events and customs, and itself shapes the narratives of experiences. Included within this realisation, is the fact that although phenomenology is concerned with structures of consciousness and experiences that we have as conscious beings, these structures are often dependent on the context in which they operate. As such, although informative, the phenomenology of, for instance, loss and grief in isolation from their sociocultural context, remains abstract and incomplete. It is only when experiences are considered as situated in a context, shaped by the values and norms accepted by those who dwell in the context, that the experience and its significance can be fully apprehended and appreciated. It is due to the realisation of this importance that, throughout the work, I have aimed to emphasise the role of culture in shaping experiences and show how variations in experiences of depression can be explained through cultural considerations.

Secondly, the realisation that multiple factors have an influence on shaping the world of experiences, leads to certain methodological difficulties. This is since, depending on the lens through which the experiences are investigated and narratives interpreted, different pictures of the experiences emerge. In attempting to understand experiences of depression in Iran, there are different points of emphasis. For instance, the image presented in this work is based on the cultural frames of thought, as seen particularly in religious modes of understanding, and works of literature. In contrast, Behrouzan (2016) focuses on understanding *depreshen* in the context of generational memories of a certain point in time. Other works could aim to understand depression and experiences of it in Iran, with different points of focus and emphasis, potentially yielding different results. This is not to say that each of these analyses is incomplete and lacking substance in some way. On the contrary, I would argue that these should be viewed as complementary: it is only through examining the phenomenon and experiences of it from different perspectives that a more complete image can start to emerge. In other words, due to the multidimensionality of experiences as situated within a complex context, the way experiences of a phenomenon such as depression are to be understood and interpreted can take various forms depending on the focus on a particular dimension of the significance of experiences.

The Problem of Interpretation and Idioms of Distress

An investigation such as the present one, whose starting point is first-person reports of experiences, is no stranger to the problem of interpretation. Such a study, on the one hand is praised for going back to the first-hand experience of individuals and taking those individual expressions and experiences seriously, while on the other hand being criticised for lacking generalisable maxims with demonstrable truths. How ought we to take such first-person accounts at face value, as true significators of underlying experiences, while simultaneously acknowledging that the experience of depression affects one's perceptions of oneself and her world in fundamental ways?

The overarching aim of a cross-cultural phenomenological study is revealing broad principles and frameworks that affect our experiences of a phenomenon. In this sense, individual understandings, narratives, and interpretation of the phenomenon take precedence over underlying experiences that are individually interpreted. Recall the example of grief experiences across cultures—in the absence of phenomenological isomorphism and access to one's experiences, personal narratives as situated within a significative cultural context are all that can be known and studied. Indeed, a phenomenon may be experienced by individuals in any number of ways but what ties these experiences together is the shared language and context that give the experience meaning and significance. Iranians often point to environmental factors beyond their control and a general sense of dissatisfaction as causing, or at least contributing to their depressive experiences. This is, however, expressed in different ways that could be interpreted differently if taken at face value, with the literal meaning taken as the intended meaning, or metaphorically, sarcastically, or as a joke.

#13(M) – I think [the cause of my depression is] the inability to communicate with the opposite sex, not having sex, not having a job relevant to my subject and specialisation, the frayed clothes, so that [I] can't leave the house too much, being mocked by other people, others talking behind one's back and different [malicious] labels attached to one (spook, womanizer, extremist ...), unresolvability of the socio-political problems, the falling and burning of Plasco [an iconic building in Tehran], not having money to do what others do, my computer being old and shattered, not having a smart phone and spending more time at a computer which always has to have a fan next to it, my father's poverty, the barbarity of Hezbollah, and extreme hair loss.

Given this complexity and the different modes of interpretation in the face of methodological difficulties, the question arises as to how these reports ought to be understood. Some theorists have suggested that they should be classified as 'idioms of distress'. The notion is often used in cases where a symptom report is closely tied to cultural expressions and modes of communications. Mark Nichter first defined the concept based on the following observation:

> In any given culture a variety of ways exist to express distress. Expressive modes are culturally constituted in the sense that they initiate particular types of interaction and are associated with culturally pervasive values, norms, generative themes, and health concerns. (Nichter 1981, p. 279)

Nichter argues that by viewing "ethnopsychiatric phenomena as idioms of distress", greater perspective and better understanding can be facilitated, through the recognition of the complex systems of thought and meaning in different cultures that underlie conceptualisations of phenomena. Thus, idioms of distress denote "socially and culturally resonant means of experiencing and expressing distress in local worlds" (Nichter 2010, p. 405). These are varied based on the cultural traditions of understanding human distress, as well as culturally specific ways of conveying experiences (e.g. metaphors in language, and folk theories of medicine).

The notion is closely connected with that of culture-bound syndromes, which originally designated the varied phenomena in different cultures as the variations of the universal categories of psychiatric disorders, such as schizophrenia or depression (Yap 1969). Nichter saw idioms of distress as a more befitting characterisation than syndromes per se. On his account, different sickness categories each describe "local reactions to particular forms of psychiatric distress that arise in the differing situations of disparate cultures. Some of these ways of expressing distress become formalized with names in local languages, but do not necessarily become as rigidly defined as are psychiatric diagnoses" (Rebhun 2004).

Different authors employ the concept of 'idioms of distress' in different ways. Sometimes 'idioms of distress' are taken to be cultural illness syndromes (e.g. Brain Fag Syndrome affecting West African students (Ebigbo et al. 2015)), and psychological and/or somatic complaints (e.g. reports of pain (Keyes and Ryff 2003)), which signify variations in the manifestations and articulations of distress and suffering. This is while for other authors 'idioms of distress' are the systems of beliefs, values, and cultural norms, which underlie the cultural ways of encountering and interpreting distress, as well as the way these experiences are framed and manifested in behaviour. Such idioms include religious involvement, attribution of one's state to witchcraft assault, and acting-out behaviours (Hinton and Lewis-Fernández 2010). Despite its broad use in the literature, I claim that the notion of idioms of distress does little by way of explaining the interpretive difficulties laid out above, since it is too vague to have any explanatory power. This is especially manifest within a framework that views experiences and narratives as essentially tied with culture. An exposition of two cases where this notion has been adopted in the literature would suffice to demonstrate this point.

Khyâl attacks as an example of culture-bound syndrome have been recorded in parts of Asia, particularly the South East. *Khyâl* is conceptualised as "a pathological windlike substance, a substance often described by the same local word for external winds … [and] is thought to cause havoc in the body and to potentially cause death" (Hinton et al. 2010, p. 245). Khyâl attacks sometimes resemble symptoms seen in malaria. In a study on Cambodian refugee populations, Khyâl attacks are seen as closely linked with panic attack and PTSD symptoms, and are often generated by trauma, and are thought to represent a case of "how trauma results in certain somatic symptoms in a particular cultural context" (ibid., p. 273). The association between trauma and symptoms characteristic of Khyâl attacks is such that, the authors argue, "enacting the malarial episode has become an idiom of distress and a key shaper of the anxiety experience, a key anxiety-related cultural syndrome" (ibid., p. 267). But it is not just the malarial symptoms characteristic of Khyâl attacks that represent an idiom of distress (or a cultural syndrome) in this case, as the authors argue that the attacks themselves should be understood as such. They argue that Khyâl attacks, as presented in their study, represents an instance of an idiom of distress "that has great overlap with panic attacks, panic disorders, and PTSD" (ibid., p. 273).

Khyâl attacks present a case where idioms of distress are construed as closely connected with (if not equivalent to) cultural syndromes, and representing a culturally specific manifestation of PTSD, a DSM-defined disorder. The authors argue that Khyâl attack as explored in their study, "is one of several ethnobehavioral pathways that are available when feeling distressed, is one culturally determined dysphoria form among many others" (Hinton et al. 2010, p. 275). Khyâl attacks, therefore, are understood as a cultural embodiment of negative affects, including dysphoria and anxiety, and a cultural way of both indicating distress, and responding to it. The close resemblance and association between Khyâl attacks and PTSD is further seen as evidence that Khyâl attacks are the cultural manifestation of PTSD itself; "in societies in which 'PTSD' is a known entity in the general population (it is not in the Cambodian case), the layperson's understanding of 'PTSD' may play the role of an 'idiom of distress', of cultural syndrome" (ibid., p. 276). It should be noted that Khyâl attacks are also included in the DSM-5 list of cultural concepts of distress.

The second example is the case of 'thinking too much' idioms. These idioms, rather than being unique to one culture, are seen across different cultural groups and appear in different ethnographic studies of mental distress and disorders. DSM-5 has recognised idioms of 'thinking too much' (under the equivalent term in Shona, *Kufungisisa*) as cultural explanations seen among the Shona of Zimbawe, although the description acknowledges that such expressions are used in many different cultures (American Psychiatric Association 2013, p. 834). A systematic overview of the literature on these idioms, shows that they are prevalent, to different degrees, all around the world. Although the frequency of studies done on the subject is considerably higher in Africa (43.5%) and South East Asia (29.7%), than it is in the US/Europe and Australia (2.9% each) (Kaiser et al. 2015, p. 172).

'Thinking too much' idioms, have been the subject of studies, both in their own right, and as accompanying psychiatric disorders, most often general distress and depression. Perhaps mirroring the use of this idiom by individuals and cultural groups, different studies have examined the idiom as a symptom, a syndrome, or explanation or cause of an illness, physical and psychiatric alike. These different descriptions of the idiom have not been viewed as mutually exclusive and various studies consider 'thinking too much' as belonging to two or all of the above categories. Here, then, we have a case of an idiom of distress, that (1) cannot be considered as culturally specific, as it is seen in various different cultures and geographical locations around the world, and (2) is not clearly significative of any particular element of an illness or disorder. It seems, instead, that the use of the notion of idiom of distress in this case, merely signals the fact that an expression is used widely in different cultures to convey an array of different meanings, but that is often associated with distress.

These two examples are sufficient to show the diversity in use of 'idioms of distress'. In the first case, the notion, equated with cultural syndromes, signifies a cluster of symptoms documented among a particular group of people, with considerable overlap with commonly known symptoms of panic attacks and PTSD. In the second case, the category of 'idioms of distress' is applied to an expression of rumination, seen in most cultures and parts of the world, thus in effect removing the cultural specificity of the notion. The notion is also more ambiguous in the second case, as it is not clear what it signifies and to which conditions it applies.

The variation in the use and application of 'idioms of distress' can in part be attributed to the different aims and points of interest related to the notion in the literature. For instance, some scholars argue for the use of the notion with the aim of improving clinical care and to emphasise the importance of understanding patients' cultural background that play a role in their symptomatology (e.g. Hinton and Lewis-Fernández 2010). The notion has indeed been useful and informative in these areas, as well as in reducing stigmas (e.g. Kohrt and Hruschka 2010), and developing and adapting local assessment tools for care and research (e.g. Weaver and Kaiser 2015). Despite its clinical implications, it remains unclear whether the notion signifies 'real' psychiatric categories. As Hacking has noted in his discussion of fugue, certain categories of mental illnesses are unique to a certain context and disappear once the conditions of the context changes (Hacking 1998). Hacking uses the notion of 'ecological niches' to argue that a certain cultural context (including norms and customs as well as historical and/or folk conceptualisations) at a certain point in time can give rise to and accommodate a category of mental illness, especially those that fit in an already existing medical taxonomy (note the similarities drawn between Khyâl attacks and PTSD). Yet with changing circumstances, including the changes in what the psychiatric consensus of the day consider as constituitive of a disorder, the previously identified categories of mental illness may disappear, as did hysterical fugue. Thus one problem with the notion of idioms of distress, in its clinical interest and application, is the fact that they could be signifying such 'transient mental illnesses': "an illness that appears at a time, in a place, and later fades away" (Hacking 1998, p. 1).

Other scholars are interested in other elements revealed through the notion. In particular, various anthropologists have noted that "idioms of distress can communicate suffering that does not reference psychopathological states, instead expressing collective and social anxiety, engaging in symbolic protest, or providing 'metacommentary on social injustice'" (Kaiser et al. 2015, p. 171). Understanding the notion in these terms, would in turn shift the focus to questions regarding power (who defines distress?), and away from cultural understandings of health and illness, which were the focus of the original definition given by Nichter.

With this exposition in mind, it could be suggested that pain reports among the Iranian depressed patients should be classified as an instance of idioms of distress. This is especially the case since one way of understanding pain reports in Iran is as a proxy for the expression of being in distress, as a result of too much work and responsibility, or general stress. Such an understanding is in line with accounts arguing that reports of physical distress can be thought of as idioms of distress, especially in cultures where "somatizing indirectly expresses, and is understood by others as, emotional distress" (Keyes and Ryff 2003, p. 1833). However, this is not the only symptom among Iranian patients that can be characterised as an idiom of distress. Rather, given the way the notion has been defined and used in the literature, many of the symptoms discussed in this work, such as aggressive behaviours and hostility towards others, might be considered as 'idioms of distress'. Potentially, given the link between various symptom reports and the general dissatisfaction with the conditions under which the society is organised and operates, and given the role of cultural understanding and conceptions in experiences and narratives of depression, depression itself might be construed as an idiom of distress. In this sense, depression would be used as an umbrella term and a framework, within which individuals express and understand their experiences, particularly of distress. Behrouzan's account of *depreshen* is an example in this regard, with a group of individuals "choosing a clinical language to express [their] emotional state. The psychiatric vernacular has helped [them] situate [their] present-day emotional distress within historical and social contexts" (Behrouzan 2016, p. 93). This would be especially the case for those who, rather than having received a formal diagnosis of depression, self-identify as such.

These examples show that the notion of idioms of distress is useful only insofar as it signifies the interconnectivity of cultural conceptions with narratives and experiences of phenomena, as laid out above. Since cultural modes of thought and understanding are pervasive in everyday conceptualisations and narratives of experiences, any form of cultural variation in experiences and articulations of psychiatric disorders can be classified as an idiom of distress. Such a classification, however, does not, and cannot explain the significance of this interconnectivity and its influence on experiences. In other words, talk of idioms of distress indicates *that* culture influences narratives and experiences of illness, without showing *how* this is done. Within a theoretical framework that asserts a fundamental inseparability between experiences, narratives, and cultural scripts and modes of understanding, it is difficult to isolate a single element as giving rise to a particular experience. Therefore, an unshakable interpretation, in the sense of a clear-cut mapping and categorizing of experiences and reports onto cultural frameworks, remains an elusive task.

9

Concluding Remarks

This project set out to answer particular questions regarding cross-cultural variations in experiences of depression, as seen in Iran and the UK. As the empirical data suggests, such variations can be seen in the presence of particular symptoms and absence of others, as well as in the variations in the emphasis placed on different symptoms. Iranians, unlike patients in the UK, rarely complain of having feelings of guilt in depression, and instead present with aggression and aggressive behaviour. Patients in the UK complain of feeling lonely and isolated in depression, whereas those in Iran talk about a tendency and desire towards isolation. Whilst hopelessness is present in both samples, the emphasis placed on this feeling among the Iranian population is much stronger. Hopelessness among Iranian patients is accompanied by feelings of absurdity, which highlight the loss of meaning, rather than sadness, as the central complaint in depression. There have, of course, also been similarities between the complaints and symptom reports, such as the embodied experience of depression manifested in the perception of one's body as heavy and leaden, and the perception of time as slowing down in depression. These similarities and differences have been accounted for within the unique sociocultural context in which they arise.

M. Mirdamadi, *A Phenomenological Study of Depression in Iran*,
https://doi.org/10.1007/978-3-031-30407-1_9

Throughout the analysis, the individuals and their experiences are viewed as situated within a phenomenologically significant world, thus enabling an analysis that takes culture as a central influencing factor. Within this phenomenological outlook, a close examination of some of the important pillars of Iranian culture and observation of forces that shape the dominant discourse in the country today, have informed the analyses. As such, the discussions and argument here trace the different manifestations and articulations of depression to pre-existing cultural frames of thought and interpretation, which underlie the variations seen in experiences of depression. In this context, cultural conceptualisations of life, health and illness, cultural ways of relating to the world and other people, and cultural ways of thinking about life and death, have been shown to play an important role. As I have argued, many of these cultural frameworks for thought, understanding and interpretation, although pervasive in all aspects of life, remain largely unconscious. This is indeed not surprising, given the fact that they are internalised through years and centuries of practice, and their influence on the way a phenomenon is experienced and articulated is only revealed through a close examination of the network of cultural meaning-making mechanisms.

The contribution of this work to the body of literature on cross-cultural variations in mental disorders lies in its outlook; not only does it aim at recording the variations as they are seen between different sociocultural contexts, but it also attempts to give an account of the roots of such variations, tracing them in their cultural and historical trajectory. In this sense, the arguments presented here lay out not only the fact of the matter that there are such variations across cultures, but also the ways through which these variations can be made sense of and understood. Importantly, the analyses given here aim to recognise the different historical, political and ideological, linguistic, as well as cultural elements that together shape the background of experiences and form the mechanisms through which cultural variations in experiences arise.

In the previous chapter, I offered some theoretical implications of the thesis for the way we understand experiences, and how these are inseparable from the cultural context in which they are had, as well as from the narratives that express them. But the arguments presented throughout this work have broader implications for psychiatry as a science and practice. In particular, they raise a question as to what ought to be considered a psychiatric symptom rather than a non-pathological reaction to the goings-on in one's world and environment. As a consequence of this problem, we are then faced with the issue of what it means to have a universal criterion for a psychiatric disorder such as depression. Furthermore, the preceding arguments have an implication for phenomenology as a theory and method. For accepting that experiences are fundamentally cultural, as I argued in the previous chapter, means redefining the subject matter of phenomenological investigation and consequently the methodology adopted for it. I will look at each of these in turn.

Implications for Psychiatry

A central claim in this work has been that culture, as a system of values and customs, but also of thoughts and interpretation, has a considerable role in shaping manifestations and experiences of depression. The way in which this role is played is through the influence of cultural modes of thought on the conceptualisations of phenomena, which in turn shape the way a phenomenon is experienced. Accepting this mechanism raises questions about the way we commonly think about psychiatry and our expectations of its practice. If it can be established, as I have argued, that various external factors including culture and society can, in large part, shape psychiatric illnesses, then the status of psychiatry as a science that sets out to investigate mental disorders assumed to take much the same form across cultures is undermined.

The criteria for defining and diagnosing mental disorders, as set out by the *Diagnostic and Statistical Manual of Mental Disorders* (DSM), assumes that the manifestation and articulation of depression, bar some negligible differences, remain largely similar and identifiable regardless of the cultural context in which they are experienced and observed. As the discussions in this and other works show, however, common symptoms of depression can differ across cultures, in ways that do not necessarily represent the DSM criteria. Related to the concern regarding diagnostic criteria is the question of what should be considered a symptom at all. As the discussions on idioms of distress in Chap. 8 show, there are blurred lines between what is considered pathological, and what is merely an accepted way of talking about distress and dissatisfaction in a given culture and society. Such blurred lines have implications for what can plausibly be considered a symptom of a pathological state in a given sociocultural context. Furthermore, in considering these blurred lines we are ultimately confronted with the question of where a disorder resides; in few individuals in a society, as is often presumed, or could there be a point where a society as a whole can be thought to be 'disordered'? I will not attempt to answer here whether or not a 'disordered society' can be made sense of, but instead, I will illustrate the circumstances under which this question arises.

The sociocultural context at a given point in time has a clear bearing on where the line separating a pathological symptom from a normal reaction to environmental stressors is drawn. For instance, hopelessness is one of the important elements in the identification and diagnosis of depression, and as has been seen, represents one of the most important elements of experience of depression in Iran. The problem of hopelessness in Iran, however, is not limited to depression, and rather, has been viewed as one of the most pressing sociological crises facing the country (Center for Strategic Studies 2018). In the last decade, due to political and economic issues in Iran, and notably due to lack of change, hopelessness has increased among Iranians regardless of their situation in the society. The high prevalence of hopelessness in Iranian society has initiated various debates, some of which conflate socio-political hopelessness, as seen on a social level, with psychological hopelessness seen on an individual level. Such viewings in turn have led to debates which resort to explain the socio-political situation with the help of medical, in particular psychiatric, nomenclature. These debates are often centred around the question of whether Iranian society as a whole can be considered to suffer from depression (e.g. Pargar 2017), thus arguably portraying depression as an inevitable state, not of any single individual, but of the society that encompasses the world of many individuals. This inevitability of depression is seen repeatedly in the respondents' view of what depression is, and what they view to be the causes of their own depression. In such cases, the conflation of various forms of hopelessness, and especially the explanation of socio-political hopelessness in terms of depression further blurs the line between what is considered to be pathological and what is a normal, albeit unpleasant and problematic, state of the world and one's position within it.

Similarly, complaints of feelings of absurdity and aggressiveness towards other people can be shown to be, in part, a normalised presence in Iranian society, rooted in the socio-political shortcomings which exacerbate a sense of helplessness and frustration among people. Given the prevalence of hopelessness, which is in large part due to people's inability to bring about change, and which prevents individuals from being able to imagine a good future for themselves, one can expect to see a sense of despair among the population. In this sense, given the impossibility of change, the continuation of life can strike one as absurd and frustrating. Such feelings, in their external expression, could easily be manifested in the form of aggressive behaviour. As Kashi has noted, there are fundamental differences between the different forms of complaints, those made on a daily basis encompassing the everyday life of Iranians, and those which designate a pathological issue, as they arise due to different and often distinct circumstances. "In the circumstances of the [Iranian] society today, if we view the [socio-political] projects promised after the revolution as failed, it would mean, either that we encounter a society suffering from lack of meaning, in itself a political matter, or that we encounter a fatigued and angry society, which is again a political matter" (Kashi 2018—my translation). Viewed in this way, it can be seen that these symptoms rather than signifying psychological problems that could be construed as pathological, and treatable through medication, can be thought to be a normal reaction to the socio-political difficulties.

The problem here is that often there are no obvious ways of separating these various complaints. Such a difficulty can lead to complications for psychiatrists and mental health professionals, since it is the totality of individuals' experiences, political, cultural, and pathological alike, which together shape narratives of depression among Iranians. This difficulty is due to *structuring*, i.e. "the ways sociocultural factors shape generalized distress into particular outcomes" (Horwitz 2002, p. 114), which may or may not be in line with psychiatric diagnostic criteria. Structuring brings under question the assumption of diagnostic psychiatry—that particular symptom clusters denote a specific underlying disease entity—since as has been shown throughout this work, symptom reports are inseparable from the context in which they are expressed. One could expect, for instance, that the complaints rooted in socio-political difficulties could 'spill over' to complaints considered pathological by a specialist. This expectation is further strengthened given the often fuzzy line between what is considered pathological and what has become a normal, routine way of expressing dissatisfaction and distress in the broader sociocultural domain. Furthermore, the dominant discourse present in the society, rather than aiming to explain and separate these elements, either dismisses, or frames the socio-political complaints in medical terms—as is seen in the increasing number of discussions on depression, not as a psychiatric illness, but as a sociological state of the nation.

Such descriptions of the society and its ailments, which conflate the individual and pathological, with the social and everyday normal reactions, are problematic. This is because, as the dominant discourse, they can figure into individuals' descriptions and understanding of themselves, as suffering from psychiatric disorders by virtue of being part of a society that has long manifested and experienced feelings and behaviours on the borderline of normality and pathology. As Hacking has extensively argued, descriptions of the self or of different phenomena, have a determining influence on behaviours and experiences, and on possibilities of action (Hacking 2002). Such medicalised self-descriptions and narratives could in turn pose problems when it comes to diagnosis of depression, as they are always already constructed in medical terms, determining individuals' expectations and help-seeking behaviour with regards to psychiatric professionals.

Although it is undeniable that the socio-political status of a country and the dominant discourse influence articulations and conceptualisations of depression, it is important to distinguish these influences from the cultural ones. The symptoms and behaviours that arise in a certain socio-political state can be thought of as reactions to difficulties in this domain, and thus dependent on the context of one's experience in the here and now. In contrast, the behaviours and modes of thought brought about through culture are seen as longer lasting, ones that are not readily removed with a change in the state of the one's environment and socio-political status. Descriptions that arise in a certain socio-political environment seem more prone to change, "some dropping in, some dropping out" of the collective understanding, thus changing some of the behaviours and articulations relating to them (Hacking 2002, p. 48). For instance, although the high emphasis on feelings of hopelessness could be lessened following an improvement in the socio-political state of Iran, the importance of loss of meaning as rooted in cultural conceptualisation of life, may not be altered with such a change. Of course, it should be acknowledged that cultural modes of thought are remade in light of social and political change, but an exposition of the relationship between the two would be beyond the scope of this work. It should be noted, however, that although the focus of this work has been on the influence of culture, one that has defined the modes of understanding spanning hundreds of years, conducting the present research has coincided with unprecedented socio-political turmoil in Iran, which inevitably has influenced at least part of the narratives and understandings of depression.

The particular question regarding difficulties in diagnosis is, if individuals articulate their experiences and complaints in accordance with the way depressive symptoms and depression in general are portrayed in the dominant discourse, then how ought psychiatrists to view and regard the complaints presented by individuals. For example, would the sense of hopelessness and despair be considered a symptom of depression, or merely another expression of dissatisfaction with the world one inhabits? One way of answering this problem in practical terms, may be to have culturally specific cost-benefit analysis which could guide the diagnostic and treatment processes. For instance, practitioners may judge antidepressants to be suitable only for those individuals that score a certain point on a hopelessness scale, and not for those who score a lower point. In such a scenario, the pragmatic considerations of the effectiveness and value of treatment attempts would be judged based on the severity of the symptoms, while bypassing the conceptual difficulty of determining what is to be considered pathological. Such pragmatic solutions could help minimise mistakes and over-diagnosis and overmedication, especially in cases where there are no straightforward ways of separating common ways of reporting distress and dissatisfaction from those reports that more closely resemble symptoms of depression. Although such solutions could offer practical help in such problematic cases, the need for the development of such tools also signals the shortcomings of the current available diagnostic criteria, due to their rigidity and the resulting inability to account for cultural factors that influence the manifestations of mental disorders.

The DSM criteria has been revised in light of the body of scholarly work on cross-cultural variations of mental disorders. DSM-5 indeed holds that culture, defined as "systems of knowledge, concepts, rules, and practices that are learned and transmitted across generations" (American Psychiatric Association 2013, p. 749), plays a fundamental role in shaping individuals' illness experience. The provision of Cultural Formulation, introduced in DSM-IV, and expanded on in DSM-5, aims to highlight the importance of culture, by aiming to discern, among other factors, the individuals' cultural identity, cultural conceptions of distress and illness, and common sociocultural stressors (ibid., pp. 749–760). Additionally, there are cultural provisions and complications that are acknowledged in the context of particular disorders. For instance, within the criteria for Major Depressive Disorder (MDD) in DSM-5, culture-related issues are acknowledged, albeit briefly. It is noted that cross-cultural studies of depression point to some variations, yet these do not yield culturally specific symptoms for depression, but rather indicate different emphases on particular symptoms:

> While these findings suggest substantial cultural differences in the expression of major depressive disorder, they do not permit simple linkages between particular cultures and the likelihood of specific symptoms. Rather, clinicians should be aware that in most countries the majority of cases of depression go unrecognized in primary care settings and that in many cultures, somatic symptoms are very likely to constitute the presenting complaint. (American Psychiatric Association 2013, p. 166)

In a sign of sensitivity to the workings of cultural mechanisms in shaping manifestations and experiences of mental disorders, DSM-5 proposes the use of Cultural Formulation Interview (CFI). An individual concerned with having depression may be asked whether certain elements from their cultural "background or identity" could make a difference to their depression, or cause difficulties and concerns in dealing with their depression (American Psychiatric Association 2013, p. 753). Although a welcome gesture, the arguments presented in this work demonstrate that such tools are far from effective. For although cultural frameworks can be shown to influence manifestations, articulations, and experiences of depression, these mechanisms most often operate below the surface of any individuals' consciousness. As such, attempts to discern such cultural workings from the individual patients themselves would be ineffective. It would be implausible to think that individuals may be able to answer such questions in a way that elucidates the different cultural mechanisms and dynamics that shape experiences of depression in their cultural context.

As can be seen, therefore, despite various revisions and push from researchers, the DSM has remained largely oblivious to cultural variation. This obliviousness is shared, to an extent, by some researchers within Iran, who are intent upon proving that, at least in the case of Iran, the DSM criteria for depression matches nearly perfectly with the individuals' symptoms. For instance, one group of researchers in Iran conclude that "despite criticisms of the DSM-IV-TR, we found its criteria for MDD nearly enough for the studied population" (Amini et al. 2013, p. 690), barring somatic symptoms such as pain, which they observed among their sample but are not emphasised enough in the criteria. It could be argued that the use of alternative diagnostic criteria, such as the ICD, which allow different countries to adapt their diagnostic criteria to their particular cultural context, would resolve some of the worries presented here. There are, however, concerns that the role of culture in diagnosis, as laid out by the ICD, remains nebulous and ambiguous, and therefore falls short of offering comprehensive diagnostic criteria mindful of cultural influences (Alarcón 2009). In the absence of culturally nuanced diagnostic criteria, the burden remains on practitioners to separate pathological complaints from other, socially and culturally formed complaints of distress and dissatisfaction.

Similar to the case of reports of pain, a body of research that explains the differences between such reports and complaints could ensure better understanding of patients' complaints, leading to more reliable diagnoses. The need for such an approach to diagnosis, implies that the diagnostic criteria currently in use fall short of providing a comprehensive basis for the identification of depression in light of cultural variation. In other words, it is only in conjunction with awareness of the nuances of culture and society, and the way these play a role in the narratives and experiences of mental illness that the diagnostic criteria can be used effectively. In the absence of such knowledge and sensitivity, there could be a large disparity between the individuals' understanding of mental illness, and consequently their expectations from practitioners, and the views of mental health professionals and the help they can provide. What this entails, more broadly, is the fact that the practice of psychiatry, despite being construed as universally applicable, remains (or ought to remain) dependent on, and responsive to various elements that shape the narratives, manifestations, and experiences of mental illnesses. These include sociocultural elements which vary not only across cultures, but also across time in any given culture, due to shifts in values, concerns, and modes of thought that, as noted earlier, play a role in conceptualisations and therefore experiences of mental illnesses. As such, it could be suggested that sensitivity to sociocultural norms, of discourse and practice alike, ought to be part of the process of psychiatric diagnosis and treatment, not only in Iran, but more broadly in the practice of psychiatry in any cultural context.

This latter point has further implications and consequences for psychiatry as a science with a claim to universality. For if it is accepted that the manifestations of mental illnesses are influenced by sociocultural elements, and therefore knowledge of and sensitivity to these influences should complement the diagnostic criteria, then the claim to universality of science of psychiatry is undermined. This means, in effect, that contrary to the claims made by the science of psychiatry, mental illnesses are not manifested, articulated, nor experienced in the same way across cultures. One may remedy this worry by appeal to the distinction between disease and illness: mental disorders are conceptualised as disease entities which, like biological disorders, are thought to be universal across cultures, despite the variations in illness experiences. However, as the analysis presented shows, not only are both the manifestations and experiences of depression largely shaped by culture, but mental disorders are often identified through personal reports and/or changes in behaviour, both of which are, to a considerable extent, shaped by culture and environment. This leaves little room for appeal to the supposed biological underpinnings of disorders in classifying or diagnosis of the disorders. This does not necessarily imply that the project of psychiatry as a whole fails to yield satisfactory results. But it does signal the need for better accommodation of cultural variations in the science and practice of psychiatry, including in the way mental illness more broadly, as a type of illness, with different tokens as specific disorders, is conceptualised.

There are indeed similarities seen in experiences of depression in Iran and the UK, which imply that there could be a universal categorisation of depression, despite variations in other elements of experiences. Such similarities include the perception of time as slowing down, fatigue and lack of energy, disturbances to embodiment in the form of the perception of the body as heavy and leaden. An important part of experience of depression, that also seems to be universal, is the disturbance in personal relationships. As has been discussed in Chaps. 5 and 6, there are considerable differences in how such a disturbance is manifested in Iran and the UK. Yet it can be argued that the fact of existence of such disturbances is seen in the same way in both cultures, and in instances, elements such as perceived lack of empathy and even a sense of hostility towards others remain largely similar across the two cultures. What such similarities show, I would argue, is not that depression, as a category of illness is itself culture-bound, but rather, that the way depression is classified (in particular in the DSM) is too narrow to allow for cultural variation. The DSM classifications rest upon symptom clusters and are therefore based upon how a particular disorder manifests itself. Such method of classification, as noted by Hacking, ultimately defines kinds of people and mental disorders based on a set of pre-defined conditions (Hacking 1995, p. 22). Such rigidity and specificity in identifying disorders, and describing those suffering from them (Hacking 2002, p. 109), leaves little room for accommodating cultural variation.

In distressful conditions such as depression, where cultural structuring, but also socio-political pressures play a considerable role, it is important to have an understanding that acknowledges these various influences. In these cases, "classifications that view distress as broad, as continuous, and as manifest in multiple ways are more useful than the specific, discrete, and singular categories of diagnostic psychiatry" (Horwitz 2002, p. 220). An account of depression which, rather than resting on specific manifestations (e.g. sense of guilt and worthlessness), is based on what could be thought of as core elements of depression (e.g. disturbances in interpersonal relationships) which can be manifested in different ways (sense of guilt, or aggression) would present a more reliable account of what depression is. Such an account would accommodate cultural variations without undermining the validity of the category of depression itself. Such an account could further signal the need for cultural elements to be taken into account in the diagnosis, as well as the treatment of depression.

Implications for Phenomenology

The second domain where the implications of the present study can be seen, is in the field of phenomenology, as a discipline and method. Phenomenology is concerned with structures of human consciousness, as revealed through the first-person perspective. These structures are revealed through the examination of various kinds of experiences, such as perception, thought, memory, emotion, and bodily awareness among others. These different domains of experience involve what Husserl called 'intentionality', the property of directedness of our consciousness. The fact that our consciousness is always and necessarily directed towards something out there in the world, determines the basic form of our different experiences, and relation to the world we inhabit. Despite certain differences in methods of different phenomenologists, the subject of study and the assumption behind it has remained the same; the structures of our consciousness which make our conscious experiences intelligible, are universal and unique to our mode of being as conscious humans.

What the argumentation presented in this work has shown is the fact that culture—given its influence in shaping our consciousness and conscious interpretations of the world—has a role to play in phenomenological investigation of experiences. I would argue that a greater recognition of the place of culture in our conscious understanding and experience of the world, would enable a better phenomenological understanding of such experiences. Such a recognition is in line with the history and development of phenomenology and phenomenological investigations, with the likes of Heidegger and Sartre attempting to enumerate the particular ways in which social norms and cultural backgrounds influence the phenomenological significance of our experiences.

The founder of phenomenology, Husserl, at least in his earlier writings, viewed phenomenological projects as relying on abstraction of experiences and examination of experiences in isolation. The 'phenomenological reduction' that makes possible the study of a certain experience, for Husserl, means returning to the primordial mode of experiencing, which involves bracketing out the experience, and reducing the cultural world to the world of immediate experiences or *Lebenswelt*. This reduction, therefore, "leads us back to the source of the meaning and existence of the experienced world, in so far as it is experienced, by uncovering intentionality" (Schmitt 1959, p. 240). As such, for Husserl in his early writings, the subject of phenomenological investigation is experiences in isolation, with meanings associated with the experience only by virtue of it being a conscious experience. Despite such beginnings, in his later writings Husserl gave a larger importance and significance to culture as an important constituent of the *life-world*, i.e. the context within which experiences find meaning and significance. Yet this notion of life-world, important as it may be for investigating experiences, remains an abstract notion playing a role in the scientific method of abstraction-interpretation central to Husserl's phenomenology (Carr 1970). Later phenomenologists can be thought to have attempted at clarifying this notion of life-world, not as a precondition for the abstraction of experiences central to phenomenological investigations, but rather as a concrete and tangible context within which experiences are made significant and meaningful.

Heidegger's understanding of phenomenology diverges from Husserl's, in so far as it is distanced from the phenomenological reduction so central to Husserl's understanding. More precisely, although the notion of intentionality as the characteristic property of human consciousness is central for Heidegger, he defines a more inclusive framework in which to understand and examine intentionality. As shown earlier, for Heidegger, our mode of being and our everyday experiences always find meaning within the context of the world we inhabit and where we dwell. For him, "the intentional structure is present not only in the realm of consciousness, understood in terms of man's cognitive and theoretical relation to his world, but already in the whole of man's pre-cognitive awareness … Prior to any cognitive reflection there is a primordial pre-conceptual awareness through which man already understands himself as fundamentally related to his world" (Schrag 1958, p. 121). In this sense, Heidegger's notion of Dasein being 'thrown' into the world it inhabits is made sense of, since the world is always already there, shaping our different experiences and understandings of it. As such, there is a context in which experiences are had, which cannot be separated from the experiences themselves as the subject of phenomenological study.

The brief exposition of the two understandings of what the subject of a phenomenological investigation is, and what it entails, show a move towards the recognition of the context in which we experience different phenomena. In Heidegger's understanding, the world is always pre-reflectively disclosed to us, through moods and attunements, thus determining and shaping our experiences of and within the world, as well as the significance and interpretation we attach to these experiences.

As noted in the previous chapter, the arguments presented in this work imply not only that the context of experiences ought to be acknowledged and examined in a phenomenological investigation, but also that the crucial role of culture in shaping this context should not be overlooked. If it is accepted, as I have argued in Chap. 8, that experiences are fundamentally inseparable from the cultural context which gives them meaning and significance, then phenomenology as the study of experiences ought to be able to account for the influence of culture. This would mean that within phenomenological methods, unlike Husserl's conviction, experiences cannot be isolated from the context in which they occur (recall the example of experience of loss and grief noted in the previous chapter). It also means that the context recognised in phenomenological investigations ought to go further than that suggested by Heidegger, and rather than detailing the universal context of our experience of the world, such as use of tools and relations with other people, it should examine the cultural background that shape our experiences, and reveal the world to our consciousness in a particular way.

The arguments presented throughout this work indicate that culture, as a system of beliefs and understanding of the world and our place within it, is pervasive in different elements of our experiences of the world we inhabit. The universal structures of our consciousness, as the central concern of phenomenology, are revealed through the investigation of different kinds of experiences, which are shaped, to a large extent, by culture. Studying culture as that which gives a context to our experiences, as well as defining a framework through which our experiences are made intelligible and meaningful, would allow a better understanding of the experiences under examination. Furthermore, recognising the importance of culture could give a better understanding of the structures of our consciousness, by recognising that the first-person perspective through which we are conscious of the world and our lived experiences, is always already embedded within a *cultural* world. Thus our conscious experiences and interpretations of the world are not only shaped by the universal structures of our thrownness into the world, but also the cultural framework within which our consciousness is embedded, allowing us to assign meaning and significance to the world we are pre-reflectively aware of.

This interest in culture does not mean that phenomenological investigations into types of experience that we—by virtue of the kind of being that we are—live through are futile or incomplete. It rather signals the need to acknowledge the role played by culture in shaping these experiences. In order to be informative of the nuances of our conscious awareness of the world and our place within it, phenomenological theories need to be examined against different sociocultural contexts, which through enculturation shape our different experiences. If, as I have shown, our way of being-in, and relating to the world, as well as our perceptions of ourselves and our body, is shaped by the culture, and if the world in which we are thrown is itself shaped and determined by culture, then this important element ought to be considered in phenomenological investigations. It is only through the recognition of experiences and individuals, not as abstract entities, but as situated within a phenomenologically significant cultural context, that a more comprehensive account of the workings of our consciousness can be given. In this understanding, there is no single phenomenology of depression, but different phenomenologies depending on the cultural context in which experiences of depression are examined.

This suggested approach, and indeed the one defended throughout the thesis sits nicely with the increasingly influential enactive approaches to psychopathology, which emphasise as key features of the mind its dynamical, embodied, and situated character (Colombetti 2013). Such an approach, by recognising the situatedness of the individual experiencing mental disorders, aims to paint a more comprehensive picture of the meaning and significance attached to these experiences. Furthermore, this outlook can demonstrate the ways in which this significance is both shaped by, and dependent on how an individual relates to her world *by virtue of* her embodied and situated nature, and the dynamic sense-making involved in her relation to the environment (e.g. Fuchs and Schlimme 2009; Fuchs 2014; Maiese 2016). Such approaches have also included discussions on the relation between culture and experiences of mental disorder (e.g. Durt et al. 2017; Kirmayer and Ramstead 2017). As Kirmayer and Ryder have noted, psychopathology involves psychological, social and cultural processes in addition to neurological ones, and the effects of culture on psychopathology are seen "not only at the level of the nervous system but also through social structure, institutions and practices" (Kirmayer and Ryder 2016, p. 146). The present study, its conclusions and suggested future approaches therefore, aim at furthering such a multidimensional approach to the study of mental disorders and their experiences.

Psychiatry and phenomenology are both, to different extents, concerned with people, as the beings that live through conscious experiences, and as those who can be diseased and distressed. What the implications laid out for both fields reveal, is the inadequacy of a universal understanding of people and the phenomena they encounter and experience. This universal understanding views people as largely similar in how they understand, encounter and experience different phenomena, and in how different phenomena are manifested in them. The arguments presented in this work reveal the shortcomings of such an understanding, and reveal various important nuances that, although crucial, remain overlooked in this way of framing and understanding people. In order to understand human experiences and the different phenomena they encounter in their different ways, the role of culture, as an organising force for thought, interpretation, and action ought to be recognised and examined alongside other important elements. Once it is acknowledged that we, as human beings, are fundamentally cultural beings, with our experiences and interpretations of the world as always already embedded and situated within a cultural world, the importance of including culture in examinations of our behaviour in different fields of interest is made clear. It is only through this recognition of the centrality of culture that the study of people, with their normal and pathological behaviours and experiences can be made complete.

Appendix – Depression Questionnaire

The following questionnaire, alongside an information sheet and consent form, was translated into Farsi and used in the acquisition of data among the Iranian sample.

Personal Details

Age:............Sex:...................Place of residence:.................

Have you ever been diagnosed with depression? If so, please give details of your diagnosis and the type of treatment you have received.

Have you ever been diagnosed with any other mental illnesses? If so, please give details.

M. Mirdamadi, *A Phenomenological Study of Depression in Iran*,
https://doi.org/10.1007/978-3-031-30407-1

Questions

1. Describe your emotions and moods during those periods when you are depressed. In what ways are they different from when you are not depressed?
2. Does the world look different when you're depressed? If so, how?
3. Do other people, including family and friends, seem different when you're depressed? If so, how?
4. How does your body feel when you're depressed?
5. How does depression affect your ability to perform routine tasks and other everyday activities?
6. When you are depressed, does time seem different to you? If so, how?
7. How, if at all, does depression affect your ability to think?
8. In what ways, if any, does depression make you think differently about life compared to when you are not depressed?
9. If you have taken medication for depression, what effect did it have?
10. Are there aspects of depression that you find particularly difficult to convey to others? If so, could you try as best you can to indicate what they are and why they are so hard to express.
11. What do you think depression is and what, in your view, caused your depression?
12. Who and/or what have you consulted in order to try to understand your depression? (E.g., medical practitioners, friends, books, internet sources, etc.).
13. How would you describe your relationships with others when you are depressed?
14. Has the reaction of others influenced your experience of depression? If so, how?
15. What distinguishes what you're feeling as depression, from other, more general forms of sadness?
16. Are there any positive aspects associated with your depression?
17. If there are important aspects of your experience of depression not covered by this questionnaire please describe them here.*

* Questions 1–12 and 17 were used by the research team at Durham University, for the *Experiences of Depression* study. The questions are available online and reproduced in publications following the study.

Bibliography

Aflakseir, A. 2014. The Reasons for Fear of Death and Religiosity with Anxiety in Students in Shiraz University (in Farsi). *Journal of Psychology (Tabriz University)* 9 (35): 19–32.

Akhavan-Sales, M. 1959. *The End of Shāhnāmeh (in Farsi)*. 1st ed. Tehran: Zaman Publications.

———. 1966. *From This Avesta (in Farsi)*. 1st ed. Tehran: Morvarid Publications.

———. 1978. *Winter (in Farsi)*. 1st ed. Tehran: Morvarid Publications.

———. 1979. *Life Says: But Again One Must Live (in Farsi)*. 1st ed. Tehran: Touka Publications.

Alamzadeh, M., and S. Rastegari. 2015. Youth Religiosity, Ideals and Facts: A Study of the Limits of Religious Discourses in the Analysis of Youth Religiosity (in Farsi). *Motale'at-e Jame'eshenakhti (Sociological Studies)* 21 (2): 159–188.

Alarcón, R.D. 2009. Culture, Cultural Factors and Psychiatric Diagnosis: Review and Projections. *World Psychiatry* 8 (3): 131–139.

Al-Issa, I. 2000. Mental Illness in Medieval Islamic Society. In *Al-Junūn: Mental Illness in the Islamic World*, ed. I. Al-Issa, 43–70. Madison, WI: International University Press.

Al-Koleini, M.i.-Y. 1990. *Osoul Al-Kafi*. Beirut: Dar-al Ta'aref al-Matbou'at.

Al-Najafi, M.H. 1984. *Jawahir al-kalam fi sharh shara'i' al-islam*. Beirut: Dar 'Ihya' al-Turath al-'Arabi.

M. Mirdamadi, *A Phenomenological Study of Depression in Iran*,
https://doi.org/10.1007/978-3-031-30407-1

Amanat, A. 2012. Iranian Identity Boundaries: A Historical Overview. In *Iran Facing Others: Identity Boundaries in a Historical Perspective*, ed. A. Amanat and F. Vejdani, 1–33. New York: Palgrave Macmillan US.

American Psychiatric Association. 2013. *Diagnostic and Statistical Manual of Mental Disorders*. 5th ed. Washington, DC; London: American Psychiatric Association.

Amini, K., R. Negarandeh, M.A. Cheraghi, and M. Eftekhar. 2013. Major Depressive Disorder: A Qualitative Study on the Experiences of Iranian Patients. *Issues in Mental Health Nursing* 34 (9): 685–692.

Ansari, N., A. Sayadani, and S. Assadi. 2012. Analysis of Semantic Dimensions of Colours in Masnavi-Ma'navi (in Farsi). *Studies in Language and Lyrical Literature* 2 (3): 21–40.

Attar, F. u.-d. 1984/1177. *The Conference of the Birds*. London: Penguin.

Avicenna, 1999/1025. *The Canon of Medicine (Al-Qanun fi al-Tibb)*. s.l.: Kazi Publications.

Bahar, M. 1997. *A Study in Iranian Mythology: First and Second Parts (in Farsi)*. Tehran: Agah Publications.

Bair, M.J., and R.L. Robinson. 2003. Depression and Pain Comorbidity A Literature Review. *Archive of Internal Medicine* 163 (20): 2433–2445.

Barzin, N. 2010. *La psychanalyse en Iran. Topique* 1 (110): 157–171.

Bateson, M.C., et al. 1977. Safā-yi Bātin: A Study of the Interrelations of a Set of Iranian Ideal Character Types. In *Psychological Dimensions of Near Eastern Studies*, ed. C. Brown and N. Itzkowitz, 257–273. Darwin Press: Princeton, NJ.

BBC Persian, 2017. *Three Mine Clearing Workers Killed and Wounded in the West Border of Iran (in Farsi)*. http://www.bbc.com/persian/iran-41756957. Accessed 30 Oct 2017.

Behrouzan, O. 2016. *Prozak Diaries: Psychiatry and Generational Memory in Iran*. 1st ed. Stanford, CA: Stanford University Press.

Bending, L. 2000. *The Representation of Bodily Pain in Late Nineteenth-Century English Culture*. Oxford: Oxford University Press.

Beytoote.com, 2015. *Floundering in the Mordāb of Depression (in Farsi)*. http://www.beytoote.com/psychology/khanevde-m/paddle3-morass-depression.html. Accessed 23 Nov 2018.

Bourdieu, P. 1977. *Outline of a Theory of Practice*. Cambridge: Cambridge University Press.

———. 1990. *The Logic of Practice*. 1st ed. Stanford, CA: Stanford University Press.

———. 1993. *The Field of Cultural Production: Essays on Art and Literature*. New York: Columbia University Press.

———. 1994. *In Other Words: Essays in Reflexive Sociology*. 1st ed. Cambridge: Polity Press.

Bourke, J. 2014. *The Story of Pain: From Prayer to Painkillers*. Oxford: Oxford University Press.

Bruner, E.M. 1986. Experience and its Expressions. In *The Anthropology of Experience*, ed. V.W. Turner and E.M. Bruner, 3–32. Urbana, IL: University of Illinois Press.

Carel, H. 2016. *Phenomenology of Illness*. Oxford: Oxford University Press.

Carpenter, S. 2000. Effects of Cultural Tightness and Collectivism on Self-Concept and Causal Attributions. *Cross-Cultural Research* 34 (1): 38–56.

Carr, D. 1970. Husserl's Problematic Concept of the Life-World. *American Philosophical Quarterly* 7 (4): 331–339.

Center for Strategic Studies, 2018. *Āyandeh pazhūhi-i Iran 96 (Iran Foresight 96)*. https://tinyurl.com/y6vwu6k6. Accessed 10 Apr 2018.

Charon, R. 2006. *Narrative Medicine: Honoring the Stories of Illness*. Oxford: Oxford University Press.

Choi, I., R.E. Nisbett, and A. Norenzayan. 1999. Causal Attribution Across Cultures: Variation and Universality. *Psychological Bulletin* 125 (1): 47–63.

Colombetti, G. 2013. Psychopathology and the Enactive Mind. In *The Oxford Handbook of Philosophy and Psychiatry*, ed. K.W.M. Fulford et al., 1083–1102. Oxford: Oxford University Press.

Corbin, H. 2014. *History of Islamic Philosophy*. London: Routledge.

Craig, K.D. 2009. The Social Communication of Pain. *Canadian Psychology* 50 (1): 22–32.

Crandell, D.L., and B.P. Dohrenwend. 1967. Some Relations Among Psychiatric Symptoms, Organic Illness, and Social Class. *The American Journal of Psychiatry* 123 (12): 1527–1538.

Dehkhoda, A.A. 1962. *Dehkhoda Lexicon (in Farsi)*. Tehran: Vajehyab.com.

Dols, M. 1992. *Majnūn: The Madman in Medieval Islamic Society*. 1st ed. Oxford: Clarendon Press.

Drehera, A., et al. 2017. Cultural Differences in Symptom Representation for Depression and Somatization Measured by the PHQ Between Vietnamese and German Psychiatric Outpatients. *Journal of Psychosomatic Research* 102: 71–77.

Durt, C., T. Fuchs, and C. Tewes, eds. 2017. *Embodiment, Enaction, and Culture: Investigating the Constitution of a Shared World*. London: The MIT Press.

Ebigbo, P.O., E.C. Lekwas, and N.F. Chukwunenyem. 2015. Brain Fag: New Perspectives from Case Observations. *Transcultural Psychiatry* 52 (3): 311–330.

Elpidorou, A. 2017. Emotions in Early Sartre: The Primacy of Frustration Andreas Elpidorou. *Midwest Studies in Philosophy* 41 (1): 241–259.

Emmons, K.K. 2010. *Black Dogs and Blue Words: Depression and Gender in the Age of Self-care*. New Brunswick: Rutgers University Press.

Encyclopaedia Iranica, 1999. *Ferdowsi, Abu'l-Qāsem*. http://www.iranicaonline.org/articles/ferdowsi-index. Accessed 7 June 2018.

Fell, J.P. 1965. *Emotion in the Thought of Sartre*. 2nd ed. New York: Columbia University Press.

Fischer, M. 1980. *Iran: From Religious Dispute to Revolution*. Cambridge, MA: Harvard University Press.

Fuchs, T. 2014. Depression, Intercorporeality, and Interaffectivity. In *Depression, Emotion, and the Self*, ed. M.R.a.A. Stephan, 183–198. Exeter: Imprint Academic Ltd.

Fuchs, T., and J.E. Schlimme. 2009. Embodiment and Psychopathology: A Phenomenological Perspective. *Current Opinion in Psychiatry* 22 (6): 570–575.

Geertz, C. 1973. *The Interpretation of Cultures: Selected Essays*. New York: Basic Books.

Ghahremani, H. 2014. *How to Treat Depression? (in Farsi)*. https://tinyurl.com/y8hklc7m. Accessed 15 Sep 2018.

Goetz, J.L., and D. Keltner. 2007. Shifting Meanings of Self-Conscious Emotions Across Cultures: A Social-Functional Approach. In *The Self-Conscious Emotions: Theory and Research*, ed. J.L. Tracy, R.W. Robins, and J.P. Tangney, 153–173. London: The Guilford Press.

Goldie, P. 2002. Emotions, Feelings and Intentionality. *Phenomenology and the Cognitive Sciences* 1 (3): 235–254.

Goldman, A.I. 2006. *Simulating Minds: The Philosophy, Psychology, and Neuroscience of Mindreading*. 1st ed. Oxford: Oxford University Press.

———. 2011. Two Routes to Empathy: Insights from Cognitive Neuroscience. In *Empathy: Philosophical and Psychological Perspectives*, ed. A. Coplan and P. Goldie, 31–44. Oxford: Oxford University Press.

Good, B.J. 1976. The Heart of What's the Matter The Semantics of Illness in Iran. *Culture, Medicine, and Psychiatry* 1 (1): 25–58.

Good, B.J., M.-J.D. Good, and R. Moradi. 1985. The Interpretation of Iranian Depressive Illness and Dysphoric Affect. In *Culture and Depression: Studies in the Anthropology and Cross-Cultural Psychiatry of Affect and Disorder*, ed. A. Kleinman and B. Good, 369–428. Berkeley, CA: University of California Press.

Hacking, I. 1995. *Rewriting the Soul: Multiple Personality and the Sciences of Memory*. Princeton, NJ: Princeton University Press.
———. 1998. *Mad Travelers: Reflections on the Reality of Transient Mental Illnesses*. Virginia: The University Press of Virginia.
———. 2002. *Historical Ontology*. Cambridge, MA: Harvard University Press.
Hafez Training and Medical Center, 2018. *Adult Neurology*. http://hafez.sums.ac.ir/index.php/1390-07-07-09-04-01/1390-07-11-05-17-51/1390-07-11-05-18-40.html. Accessed 4 June 2018.
Hall, J. 1994. *Illustrated Dictionary of Symbols in Eastern and Western Art*. Colorado: Westview Press.
Haroz, E., et al. 2016. How Is Depression Experienced Around the World? A Systematic Review of Qualitative Literature. *Social Science and Medicine* 183: 151–162.
———. 2017. How Is Depression Experienced Around the World? A Systematic Review of Qualitative Literature. *Social Science & Medicine* 183: 151–162.
Hedayat, S. 1948. *Gurūh-i Mahkūmīn va Payām-i Kafka (The Condemned Group and Kafka's Message)*. Tehran: Amirkabir.
———. 1974/1937. *The Blind Owl*. 1st ed. s.l.: Bashiri Working Papers on Central Asia and Iran.
———. 2002. *Eighty-Two Letters to Hassan Shahid-Noorayi (in Farsi)*. 2nd ed. Paris: Cheshmandaz Books.
Heidegger, M. 1962. *Being and Time*. Southampton: Basil Blackwell.
Hinton, D.E., and R. Lewis-Fernández. 2010. Idioms of Distress Among Trauma Survivors: Subtypes and Clinical Utility. *Culture, Medicine and Psychiatry* 34 (2): 209–218.
Hinton, D.E., et al. 2010. Khyâl Attacks: A Key Idiom of Distress Among Traumatized Cambodia Refugees. *Culture, Medicine and Psychiatry* 34 (2): 244–278.
Horwitz, A.V. 2002. *Creating Mental Illness*. 1st ed. Chicago, IL: The University of Chicago Press.
IASP, 2017. *IASP Terminology*. https://www.iasp-pain.org/terminology?navItemNumber=576#Pain. Accessed 10 Aug 2018.
Ibn Abi Talib, A. n.d. *Nahjul Balagha*. https://www.al-islam.org/nahjul-balagha-part-1-sermons. Accessed 23 Oct 2017.
Ilna News, 2017. The 'Blood-games' in girls' Schools Should be Taken Seriously (in Farsi). *Ilna News*, 18 January.
Jamalzadeh, A.A. 1942. *Darolmajānin*. Tehran: s.n.

Javanbakht, A., and M. Sanati. 2006. Psychiatry and Psychoanalysis in Iran. *The Journal of the American Academy of Psychoanalysis and Dynamic Psychiatry* 34 (3): 405–414.

Johnston, M. 2007. *I Had a Black Dog*. London: Constable & Robinson.

Kaiser, B.N., et al. 2015. "Thinking too much": A Systematic Review of a Common Idiom of Distress. *Social Science and Medicine* 147: 170–183.

Kamali Dehghan, S. 2014. *Iranian Pharrell Williams Fans Behind Happy Video Sentenced.* https://www.theguardian.com/world/2014/sep/19/iranian-pharrell-williams-fans-happy-video-sentenced. Accessed 18 Sep 2018.

Karamouzian, M., H. Sharifi, and A.A. Haghdoost. 2014. Iran's Shift in Family Planning Policies: Concerns and Challenges. *International Journal of Health Policy and Management* 3 (5): 231–233.

Kashi, M.G. 2018. *Political Context of the Decline in Societal Hope (in Farsi).* Tehran: Rahman Institute.

Kayali, T., and F. Iqbal. 2013. Depression as Unhomelike Being-in-the-World? Phenomenology's Challenge to Our Understanding of Illness. *Medicine, Health Care and Philosophy* 16 (1): 31–39.

Keyes, C.L., and C.D. Ryff. 2003. Somatization and Mental Health: A Comparative Study of the Idiom of Distress Hypothesis. *Social Science & Medicine* 57 (10): 1833–1845.

Kirmayer, L.J. 2001. Cultural Variations in the Clinical Presentation of Depression and Anxiety: Implications for Diagnosis and Treatment. *Journal of Clinical Psychiatry* 62 (13): 22–30.

Kirmayer, L., and M.J.D. Ramstead. 2017. Embodiment and Enactment in Cultural Psychiatry. In *Embodiment, Enaction, and Culture: Investigating the Constitution of the Shared World*, ed. C. Durt, T. Fuchs, and C. Tewes, 397–422. London: The MIT Press.

Kirmayer, L.J., and J.M. Robbins. 1991. Three Forms of Somatization in Primary Care: Prevalence, Co-occurrence, and Sociodemographic Characteristics. *Journal of Nervous and Mental Disease* 179 (11): 647–655.

Kirmayer, L., and A.G. Ryder. 2016. Culture and Psychopathology. *Current Opinion in Psychology* 8 (1): 143–148.

Kleinman, A. 1977. Depression, Somatization and the "New Cross-Cultural Psychiatry". *Social Science and Medicine* 11 (1): 3–10.

———. 1982. Neurasthenia and Depression: A Study of Somatization and Culture in China. *Culture, Medicine, and Psychiatry* 6 (2): 117–190.

———. 1986. *Social Origins of Distress and Disease: Depression, Neurasthenia, and Pain in Modern China*. New Haven, CT: Yale University Press.

Kleinman, A., and B. Good. (eds.) 1985. *Culture and Depression: Studies in the Anthropology and Cross-cultural Psychiatry of Affect and Disorder*. 1st ed. Berkeley, CA: University of California Press.

Kleinman, A., and J. Kleinman. 1985. Somatization: The Interconnections in Chinese Society Among Culture, Depressive Experiences, and the Meanings of Pain. In *Culture and Depression: Studies in the Anthropology and Cross-Cultural Psychiatry of Affect and Disorder*, ed. A. Kleinman and B. Good, 429–490. Berkeley, CA: University of California Press.

Koenig, H.G. 2009. Research on Religion, Spirituality, and Mental Health: A Review. *The Canadian Journal of Psychiatry* 54 (5): 283–291.

Kohrt, B.A., and D.J. Hruschka. 2010. Nepali Concepts of Psychological Trauma: The Role of Idioms of Distress, Ethnopsychology and Ethnophysiology in Alleviating Suffering and Preventing Stigma. *Culture, Medicine, and Psychiatry* 34 (2): 322–352.

Kövecses, Z. 2000. *Metaphor and Emotion: Language, Culture, and Body in Human Feeling*. Cambridge: Cambridge University Press.

———. 2005. *Metaphor in Culture: Universality and Variation*. Cambridge: Cambridge University Press.

Lakoff, G., and M. Johnson. 1980. *Metaphors We Live by*. Chicago, IL: University of Chicago Press.

———. 1999. *Philosophy in the Flesh: The Embodied Mind and Its Challenge to Western Thought*. New York: Basic Books.

Lakoff, G., and M. Turner. 1989. *More Than Cool Reason: A Field Guide to Poetic Metaphor*. Chicago, IL: University of Chicago Press.

Lamers, F., et al. 2011. Comorbidity Patterns of Anxiety and Depressive Disorders in a Large Cohort Study: The Netherlands Study of Depression and Anxiety (NESDA). *Journal of Clinical Psychiatry* 72 (3): 341–348.

Loeffler, A. 2007. *Allopathy Goes Native: Traditional versus Modern Medicine in Iran*. London: Tauris Academic Studies.

Lovering, S. 2006. Cultural Attitudes and Beliefs About Pain. *Journal of Transcultural Nursing* 17 (4): 389–395.

Maghsoudi, H., et al. 2004. Women Victims of Self-inflicted Burns in Tabriz, Iran. *Burns* 30 (3): 217–220.

Maiese, M. 2016. *Embodied Selves and Divided Minds*. Oxford: Oxford University Press.

Marsella, A., and G.M. White, eds. 1982. *Cultural Conceptions of Mental Health and Therapy*. Dordrecht: D. Reidel Publishing Company.

Masoodiniya, A. 2017. Hedayat Was Not a Monster, He Was Honest (in Farsi). *Vaghaye Etefaghiyeh*, 16 February.

Maton, K. 2008. Habitus. In *Pierre Bourdieu: Key Concepts*, ed. M. Grenfell, 49–66. Acumen: Durham, NC.
Mattingly, C. 1998. *Healing Dramas and Clinical Plot: The Narrative Structure of Experience*. Cambridge: Cambridge University Press.
McMullen, L.M., and J.B. Conway. 2002. Conventional Metaphors for Depression. In *The Verbal of Communication Emotions Interdisciplinary Perspectives*, ed. S.R. Fussell, 167–181. New York: Lawrence Erlbaum Associates.
McNaugher, T.L. 1990. Ballistic Missiles and Chemical Weapons: The Legacy of the Iran-Iraq War. *International Security* 15 (2): 5–34.
Merleau-Ponty, M. 2012/1945. *Phenomenology of Perception*. Abingdon: Routledge.
Minority Rights Group International, 2017. *Iran - Minority Rights Group*. http://minorityrights.org/country/iran/. Accessed 14 May 2017.
Mirdamadi, M. 2021. *Suicide in Iran; Personal Decision or Public Responsibility (in Persian)*. https://www.bbc.com/persian/blogs-55863403. Accessed July 2021.
Morton, A. 2013. *Emotion and Imagination*. Cambridge: Polity Press.
Moscoso, J. 2012. *Pain: A Cultural History*. s.l.: Palgrave Macmillan.
Mulhall, S. 1996. *Heidegger and Being and Time*. London: Routledge.
Naeem, F., M. Ayub, D. Kingdon, and M. Gobbi. 2012. Views of Depressed Patients in Pakistan Concerning Their Illness, Its Causes, and Treatments. *Qualitative Health Research* 22 (8): 1083–1093.
Najafi Ghezeljeh, T., and A.F. Hosseini. 2012. Attitudinal Barriers to Effective Cancer Pain Management (in Farsi). *Hayat (Journal of the Faculty of Nursing and Midwifery, Tehran University of Medical Sciences)* 18 (1): 89–101.
Nejati Hosseini, M. 2013. Death and Dying: Narratives in Social Science and Religious Knowledge (in Farsi). *Islam and Social Sciences* 5 (10): 37–63.
Nichter, M. 1981. Idioms of Distress: Alternatives in the Expression of Psychosocial Distress: A Case Study from South India. *Culture, Medicine and Psychiatry* 5 (4): 379–408.
———. 2010. Idioms of Distress Revisited. *Culture, Medicine, and Psychiatry* 34 (2): 401–416.
Nussbaum. M. 2001. *Upheavals of Thought: The intelligence of Emotions*. Cambridge: Cambridge University Press.
Obeydinia, M.A., and S. Valinezhad. 2009. The Comparison of Symbolic Function of 'Water' in Mystical Lyrics of Attar and Maulana (in Farsi). *Persian Literature (Baharestan Sokhan)* 12: 26–50.

Pargar, 2017. *Is There Such a Thing as a Depressed Society? [in Persian]*. https://www.youtube.com/watch?v=pWjS32oxxGs&t=5s&ab_channel=BBC Persian. Accessed June 2020.

Parker, G., Y.-C. Cheah, and K. Roy. 2001. Do the Chinese Somatize Depression? A Cross-Cultural Study. *Social Psychiatry and Psychiatric Epidemiology* 36 (6): 287–293.

Pezeshkzad, I. 2006 [1963]. *My Uncle Napoleon (Dāyi-jān Napel'on)*. New York: Modern Library.

Prinz, J. 2006. *Gut Reactions: A Perceptual Theory of Emotions*. Oxford: Oxford University Press.

Radden, J. 2003. Is this Dame Melancholy? Equating Today's Depression and Past Melancholia. *Philosophy, Psychiatry, & Psychology* 10 (1): 37–52.

———. 2009. *Moody Minds Distempered: Essays on Melancholy and Depression*. Oxford: Oxford University Press.

Ratcliffe, M. 2008. *Feelings of Being: Phenomenology, Psychiatry and the Sense of Reality*. Oxford: Oxford University Press.

———. 2015. *Experiences of Depression: A Study in Phenomenology*. 1st ed. Oxford: Oxford University Press.

Rebhun, L.A. 2004. Culture-Bound Syndromes. In *Encyclopedia of Medical Anthropology: Health and Illness in the World's Cultures*, ed. C.R. Ember and M. Ember. Boston, MA: Springer US.

Rezaeizadeh, H., M. Alizadeh, M. Naseri, and M. Shams Ardakani. 2009. The Traditional Iranian Medicine Point of View on Health and Disease. *Iranian Journal of Public Health* 38 (1): 169–172.

Richmond, S. 2011. Magic in Sartre's Early Philosophy. In *Reading Sartre: On Phenomenology and Existentialism*, ed. J. Webber, 145–160. London: Routledge.

Rumi, J. a.-D. M. 1881/1273. *The Masnavi*. London: Trübner & Co.

Ryder, A.G., and Y.E. Chentsova-Dutton. 2012. Depression in Cultural Context: "Chinese Somatization," Revisited. *Psychiatric Clinics of North America* 35 (1): 15–36.

Ryder, A.G., et al. 2008. The Cultural Shaping of Depression: Somatic Symptoms in China, Psychological Symptoms in North America? *Journal of Abnormal Psychology* 117 (2): 300–313.

Safdar, S., J.R. Lewis, and M. Daneshpour. 2006. Social Axioms in Iran and Canada: Intercultural Contact, Coping and Adjustment. *Asian Journal of Social Psychology* 9 (2): 123–131.

Samgis, B. 2016. The Busy Hour of Death (in Farsi). *Etemad Newspaper*, 23 October, p. 8.

San'ati, M. 2004. *Psychotherapy in a Death Conscious East.* http://www.mohammadsanati.net/1392/culturepsychoanalysisiran/584. Accessed 23 Oct 2017.

———. 2013. *Psychological Analyses in Art and Literature.* 6th ed. Tehran: Nashr-e Markaz Publishing Co.

———. 2015. *Sadegh Hedayat and Fear of Death: Blind Owl, Cultural History & Myth Killing, A Psychoanalytic Deconstruction.* 6th ed. Tehran: Nashr-e Markaz Publishing Co.

Sartorius, N., T.B. Üstün, Y. Lecrubier, and H.-U. Wittchen. 1996. Depression Comorbid with Anxiety: Results from the WHO Study on Psychological Disorders in Primary Health Care. *The British Journal of Psychiatry* 168 (S30): 38–43.

Sartre, J.-P. 1962. *Sketch for a Theory of Emotions.* London: Methuen & Co Ltd.

———. 2003. *Being and Nothingness.* London: Routledge.

———. 2004. *The Imaginary: A Phenomenological Psychology of the Imagination.* London: Routledge.

Schmitt, R. 1959. Husserl's Transcendental-Phenomenological Reduction. *Philosophy and Phenomenological Research* 20 (2): 238–245.

Schopenhauer, A. 1969. *The World as Will and Representation.* Vol. 1. New York: Dover Publications.

Schrag, C.O. 1958. Phenomenology, Ontology, and History in the Philosophy of Heidegger. *Revue Internationale de Philosophie* 12 (44): 117–132.

Secretariat of Council for Medical and Specialised Education - Ministry of Health and Medical Education, 2007. *Educational Programme and Terms of the Specialised Discipline of Psychiatry.* http://med.sums.ac.ir/icarusplus/export/sites/medical_school/payam/edo/download/course/ravanpezeshki.pdf. Accessed 22 June 2018.

Shoja Shafti, S. 2005. Psychoanalysis in Persia. *American Journal of Psychotherapy* 59 (4): 385–389.

Shojaeizand, A., S. Shariati Mazinani, and R. Habibzadeh Khotbeh Sara. 2006. An Analysis of the State of Religion Amongst University Students (in Farsi). *National Studies* 7 (2): 55–80.

Simon, G.E., et al. 1999. An International Study of the Relation Between Somatic Symptoms and Depression. *The New England Journal of Medicine* 341 (18): 1329–1335.

Soenke, M., M.J. Landau, and J. Greenberg. 2013. Sacred Armor: Religion's Role as a Buffer Against the Anxieties of Life and the Fear of Death. In *APA Handbook of Psychology, Religion, and Spirituality*, ed. K.I. Pargament, 105–122. Washington, DC: American Psychological Association.

Solomon, R. 2006. *Dark Feelings, Grim Thoughts: Experience and Reflection in Camus and Sartre*. Oxford: Oxford University Press.

Solomon, R.C. 1992. Existentialism Emotions and the Cultural Limits of Rationality. *Philosophy East and West* 42 (4): 597–621.

Sontag, S. 1983. *Illness as Metaphor*. London: Penguin Books Ltd.

———. 1990. *AIDS and its Metaphors*. London: Penguin Books Ltd.

Statistical Center of Iran. 2015. *Selected Results of National Consensus (in Farsi)*. Tehran: Statistical Center of Iran.

Stueber, K. 2006. *Rediscovering Empathy: Agency, Folk Psychology, and the Human Sciences*. 1st ed. Cambridge, MA: MIT Press.

Stuewig, J., and J.P. Tangney. 2007. Shame and Guilt in Antisocial and Risky Behaviors. In *The Self-Conscious Emotions: Theory and Research*, ed. J.L. Tracy, R.W. Robins, and J.P. Tangney, 371–387. New York: The Guilford Press.

Svenaeus, F. 2000a. Das Unheimliche - Towards a Phenomenology of Illness. *Medicine, Health Care and Philosophy* 3 (1): 3–16.

———. 2000b. The Body Uncanny - Further Steps Towards a Phenomenology of Illness. *Medicine, Health Care and Philosophy* 3 (2): 125–137.

———. 2011. Illness as Unhomelike Being-in-the-World: Heidegger and the Phenomenology of Medicine. *Medicine, Health Care and Philosophy* 14 (3): 333–343.

———. 2014. Depression and the Self: Bodily Resonance and Attuned Being-in-the-world. In *Depression, Emotion and the Self: Philosophical and Interdisciplinary Perspectives*, ed. M. Ratcliffe and A. Stephan, 1–16. Exeter: Imprint Academic.

———. 2015. The Phenomenology of Chronic Pain: Embodiment and Alienation. *Continental Philosophy Review* 48 (2): 107–122.

Taheri Sarteshnizi, E., and M. Moosavi. 2012. Human Awareness of Death and Meaningfulness of Life in Nahj al-Balagheh (in Farsi). *Ensanpajoohi-e Dini (Religious Anthropology)* 9 (27): 177–198.

TarikhIrani, 2014. *The Real Statistics of the War (in Farsi)*. https://tinyurl.com/y97m6nh3. Accessed 17 Oct 2017.

Tavafian, S.S., D. Gregory, and A. Montazeri. 2008. The Experience of Low Back Pain in Iranian Women: A Focus Group Study. *Health Care for Women International* 29 (4): 339–348.

Thompson. T. 1996. *The Beast: A Journey Through Depression*. New York: Plume Printing.

Thorson, J.A., and F.C. Powell. 1988. Elements of Death Anxiety and Meanings of Death. *Journal of Clinical Psychology* 44 (5): 691–701.

———. 1990. Meanings of Death and Intrinsic Religiosity. *Journal of Clinical Psychology* 46 (4): 379–391.
Triandis, H.C. 2002. Individualism-Collectivism and Personality. *Journal of Personality* 69 (6): 907–924.
Tseng, W.-S. 1975. The Nature of Somatic Complaints Among Psychiatric Patients: The Chinese Case. *Comprehensive Psychiatry* 16 (3): 237–245.
Van Ness, P.H., and D.B. Larson. 2002. Religion, Senescence, and Mental Health: The End of Life Is Not the End of Hope. *The American Journal of Geriatric Psychiatry* 10 (4): 386–397.
Vega, W.A., and R.G. Rumbaut. 1991. Ethnic Minorities and Mental Health. *Annual Review of Sociology* 17 (1): 351–383.
de Vignemont, F. 2010. Knowing Other People's Mental States as If They Were One's Own. In *Handbook of Phenomenology and Cognitive Science*, ed. S. Gallagher and D. Schmicking, 283–300. Dordrecht: Springer.
Weaver, L.J., and B.N. Kaiser. 2015. Developing and Testing Locally Derived Mental Health Scales: Examples from North India and Haiti. *Field Methods* 27 (2): 115–130.
Wollheim, R. 1999. *On the Emotions*. New Haven, CT: Yale University Press.
Wong, Y., and J. Tsai. 2007. Cultural Models of Shame and Guilt. In *The Self-Conscious Emotions: Theory and Research*, ed. J.L. Tracy, R.W. Robins, and J.P. Tangney, 209–223. London: The Guilford Press.
World Health Organization, 2018. *Latest Data on Suicide*. http://www.who.int/mental_health/suicide-prevention/en/. Accessed 15 Sep 2018.
Yap, P. 1969. The Culture Bound Syndromes. In *Mental Health Research in Asia and the Pacific*, ed. W. Cahil and T. Lin, 33–53. Honolulu: East-West Centre Press.
Ying, Y.W. 1990. Explanatory Models of Major Depression and Implications for Help-Seeking among Immigrant Chinese-American Women. *Culture, Medicine and Psychiatry* 14 (3): 393–408.
Ying, Y.W., et al. 2000. The Conception of Depression in Chinese American College Students. *Cultural Diversity and Ethnic Minority Psychology* 6 (2): 183–195.
Zarghami, M., and A. Khalilian. 2002. Deliberate Self-Burning in Mazandaran, Iran. *Burns* 28 (2): 115–119.
Zhou, X., et al. 2016. From Culture to Symptom: Testing a Structural Model of "Chinese somatization". *Transcultural Psychiatry* 53 (1): 3–23.

Index[1]

[1] Note: Page numbers followed by 'n' refer to notes.

M. Mirdamadi, *A Phenomenological Study of Depression in Iran*,
https://doi.org/10.1007/978-3-031-30407-1

FSC
www.fsc.org
MIX
Papier | Fördert gute Waldnutzung
FSC® C083411

Kolibri 360 GmbH
Ferdinand-Jühlke-Straße 7
99095 Erfurt, Deutschland
produktsicherheit@kolibri360.de